The Funny Side Collection

The Bark Side

It's a Dog's Life!

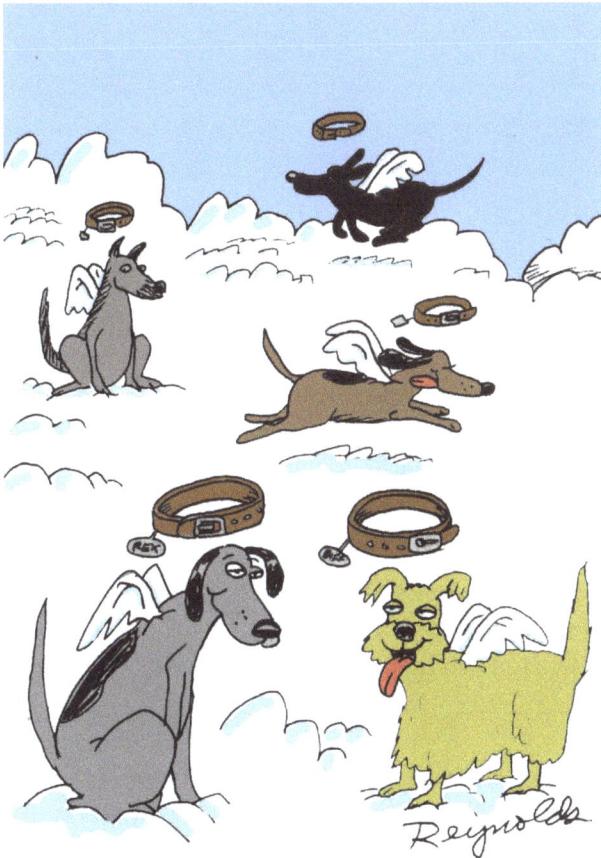

Dan Reynolds
Nancy Cetel, MD
Joseph Weiss, MD

© 2017 Dan Reynolds
　　　Nancy Cetel, MD
　　　Joseph Weiss, MD
　　　SmartAsk Books
　　　Rancho Santa Fe, California, USA
　　　www.smartaskbooks.com
　　　www.thefunnysidecoillection.com

ISBN-13: 978-1-943760-52-7 (Color Print)
ISBN-13: 978-1-943760-53-4 (e-Book)

The Bark Side: It's a Dog's Life!

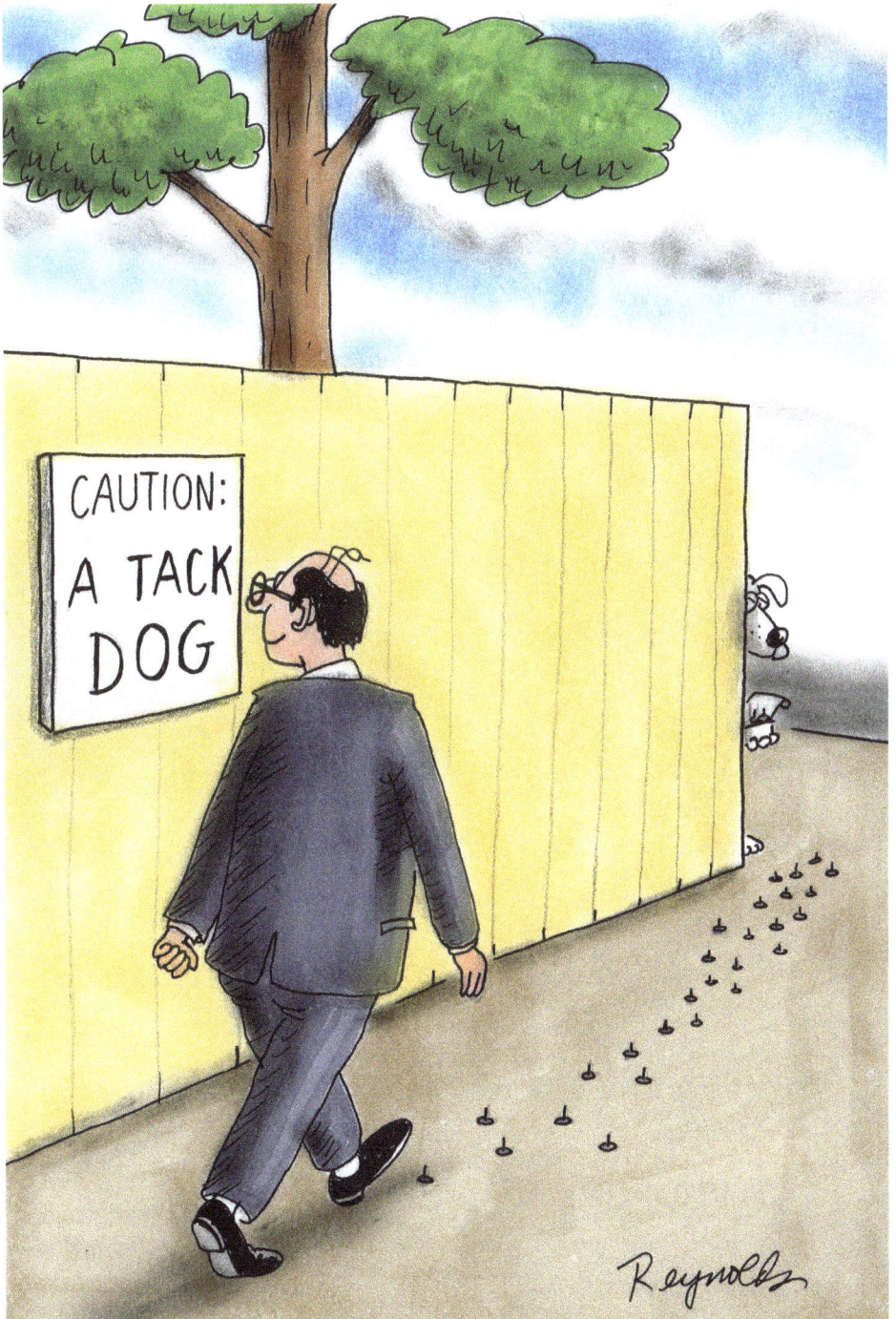

The Bark Side: It's a Dog's Life!

There are hundreds of official dog breeds in the world and even more mixes and mutts than we can count. Each dog has his own unique set of characteristics and personality. But one thing is certain – these loveable and wonderful companions are fascinating creatures.

The Newfoundland breed has a water resistant coat and webbed feet. This dog was originally bred to help haul nets for fishermen and rescuing people at risk of drowning.

Three dogs (from First Class cabins!) survived the sinking of the Titanic – two Pomeranians and one Pekingese.

It's rumored that, at the end of the Beatles song, "A Day in the Life," Paul McCartney recorded an ultrasonic whistle, audible only to dogs, just for his Shetland sheepdog.

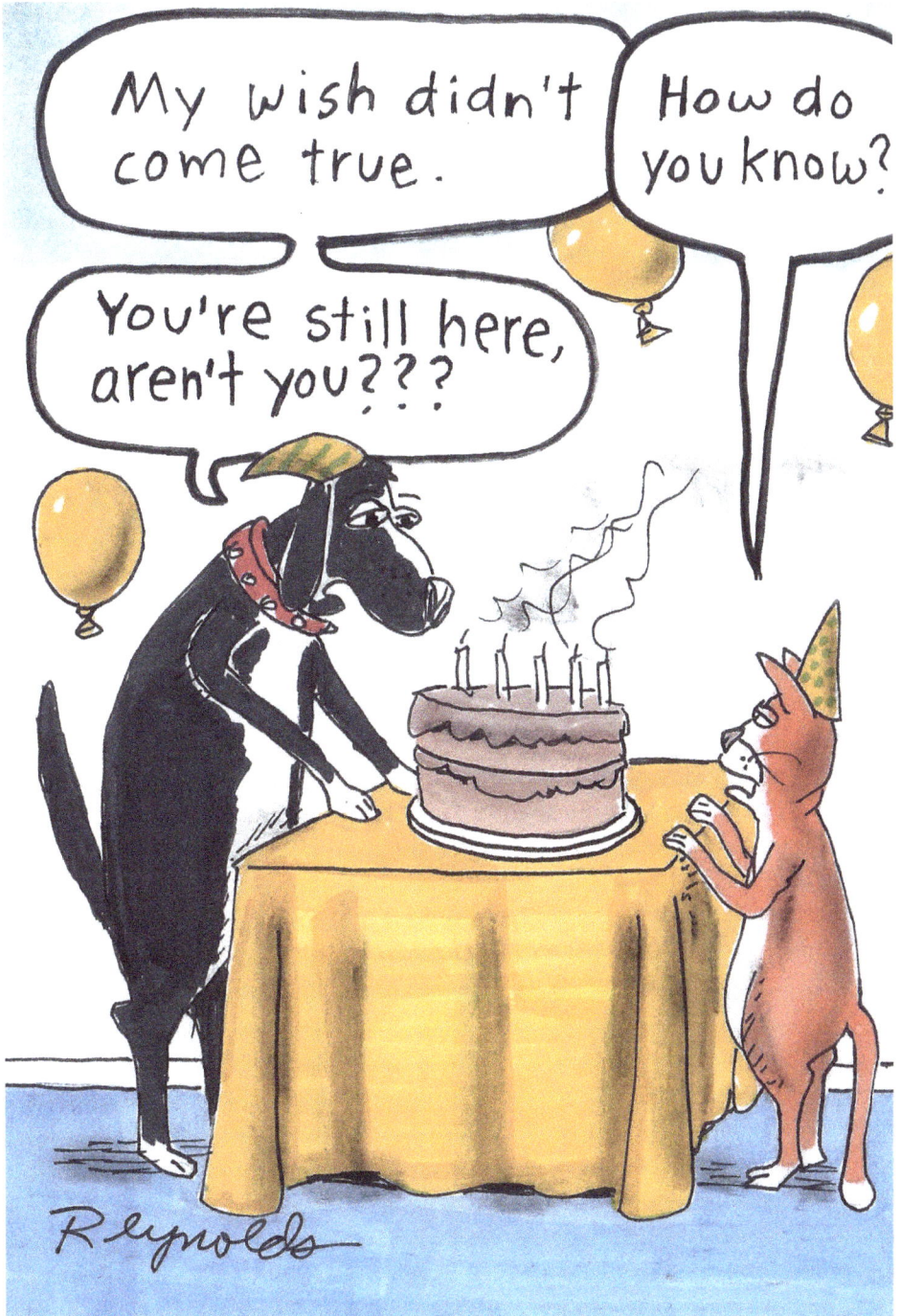

The Bark Side: It's a Dog's Life!

Dogs chase their tails for a variety of reasons: curiosity, exercise, anxiety, predatory instinct or, they might have fleas!

Dalmatian puppies are pure white when they are born and develop their spots as they grow older.

Dogs and humans have the same type of slow wave sleep (SWS) and rapid eye movement (REM) and during this REM stage dogs can dream. The twitching and paw movements that occur during their sleep are signs that your pet is dreaming

A large breed dog's resting heart beats between 60 and 100 times per minute, and a small dog breed's heart beats between 100-140. Comparatively, a resting human heart beats 60-100 times per minute.

The Bark Side: It's a Dog's Life!

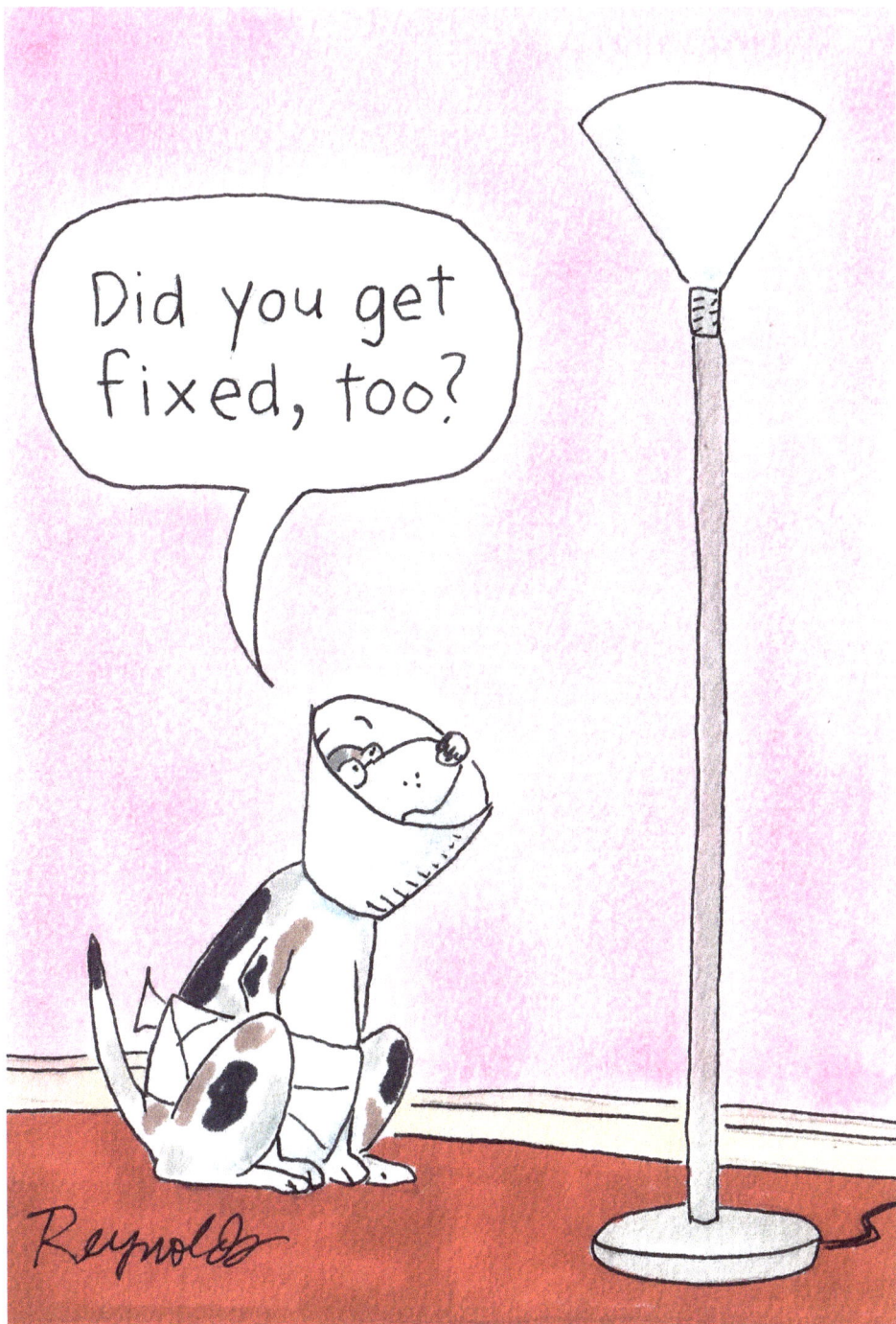

The Bark Side: It's a Dog's Life!

Dogs' eyes contain a special membrane, called the tapetum lucidum, which allows them to see in the dark.

Puppies have 28 teeth and normal adult dogs have 42.

72% of dog owners believe their dog can detect when stormy weather is on the way.

A dog's normal temperature is between 101 and 102.5 degrees Fahrenheit.

Unlike humans who sweat everywhere they have skin, dogs only sweat through the pads of their feet.

62% of U.S. households own a pet, which equates to 72.9 million homes.

45% of dogs sleep in their owner's bed (a large percentage also hog the blankets!).

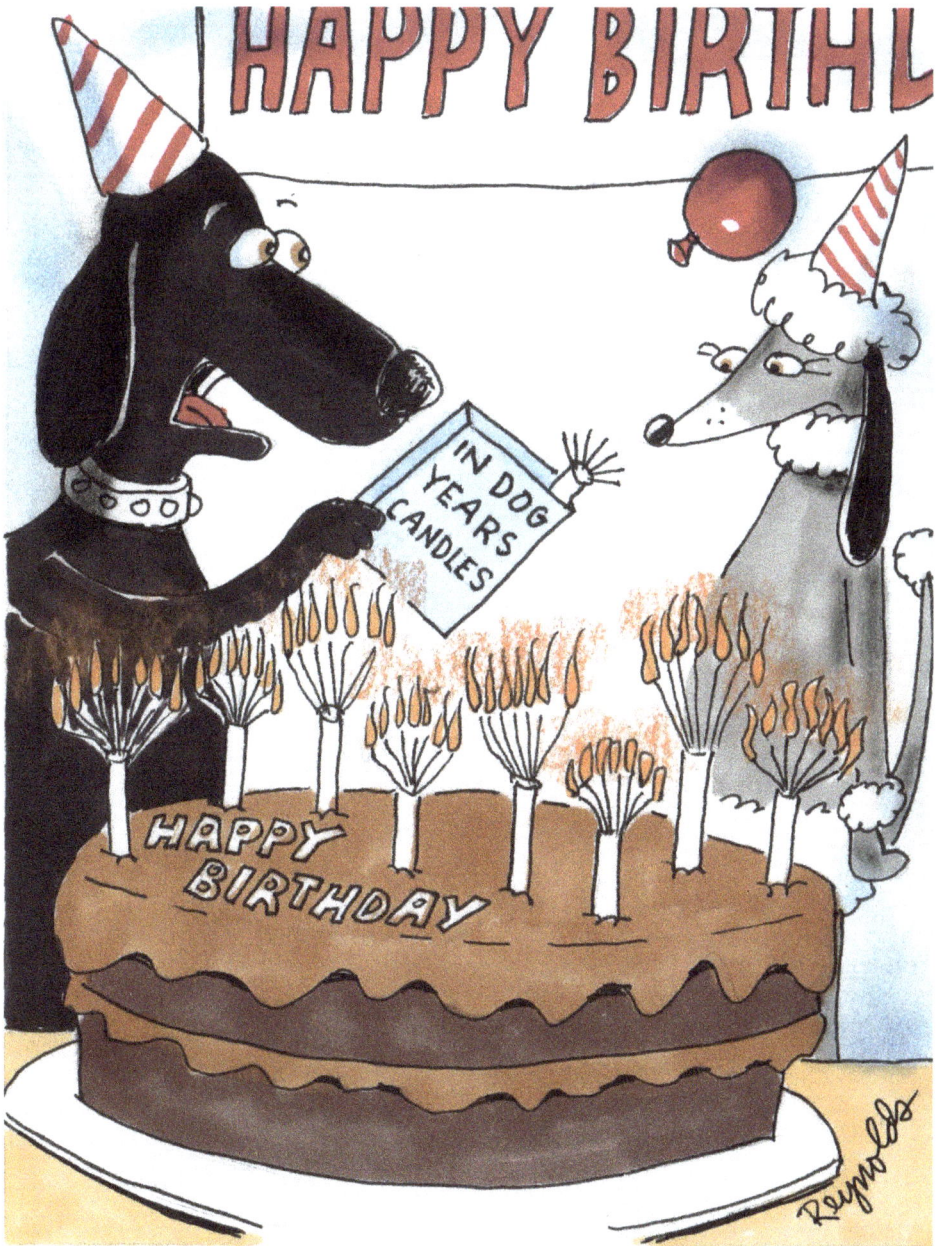

"The seven wick candles for dogs make me feel a lot older than I really am..."

Dogs' noses are wet because they secrete a thin layer of mucous that helps them absorb scent. They then lick their noses to sample the scent through their mouth.

Dogs have three eyelids, an upper lid, a lower lid and the third lid, called a nictitating membrane or "haw," which helps keep the eye moist and protected.

Dogs have about 1,700 taste buds. Humans have approximately 9,000 and cats have around 473.

It's a myth that dogs only see in black and white. In fact, it's believed that dogs see primarily in blue, greenish-yellow, yellow and various shades of gray.

Sound frequency is measured in Hertz (Hz). The higher the Hertz, the higher-pitched the sound. Dogs hear best at 8,000 Hz, while humans hear best at around 2,000 Hz.

The Bark Side: It's a Dog's Life!

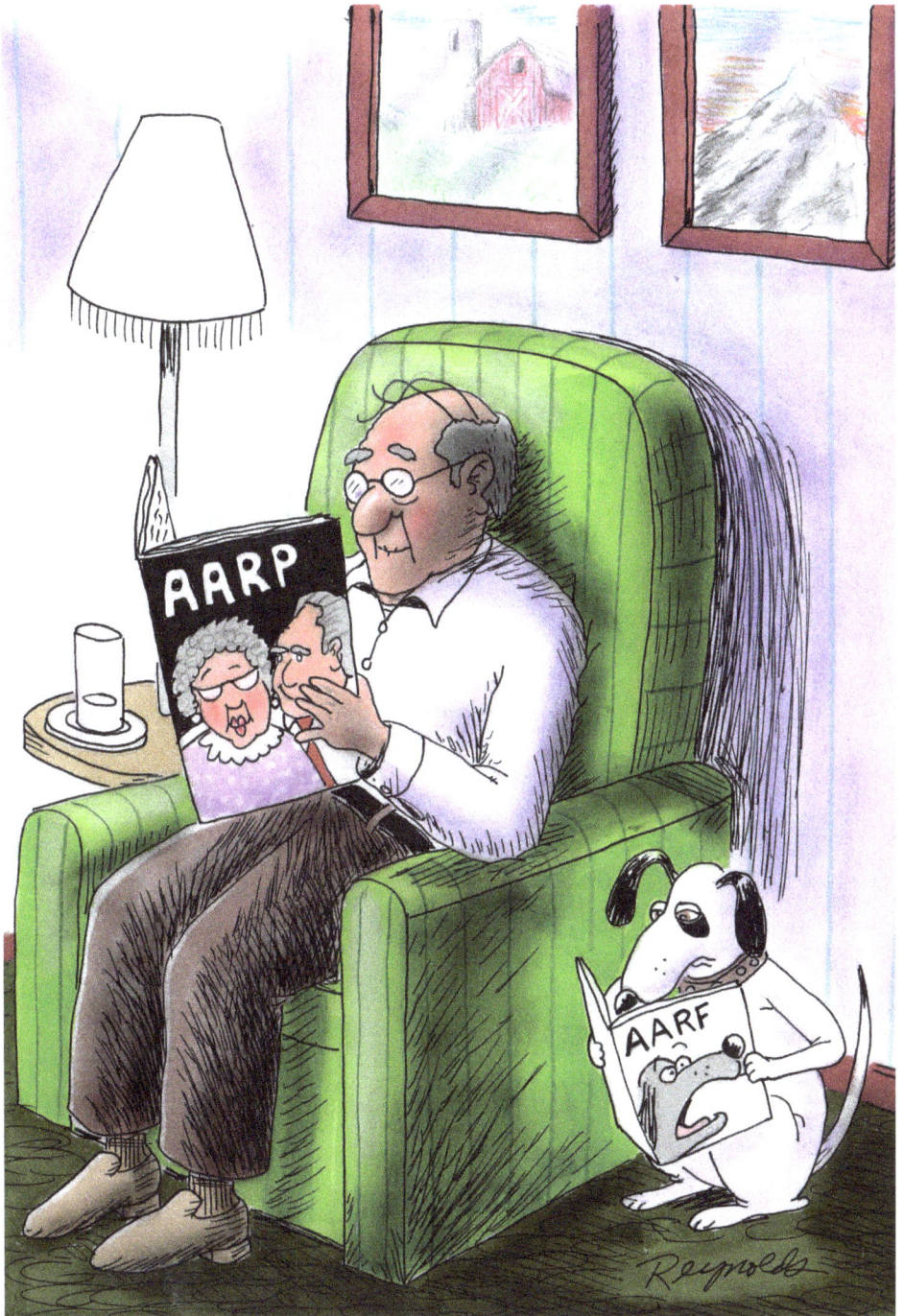

The Bark Side: It's a Dog's Life!

A Dog's sense of smell is 10,000 – 100,000 times more acute as that of humans.

Dogs' ears are extremely expressive. There are more than a dozen separate muscles that control a dog's ear movements.

While the Chow Chow dogs are well known for their distinctive blue-black tongues, they're actually born with pink tongues. They turn blue-black at 8-10 weeks of age.

When dogs kick after going to the bathroom, they are using the scent glands on their paws to further mark their territory.

Dogs curl up in a ball when they sleep due to an age-old instinct to keep themselves warm and protect their abdomen and vital organs from predators.

The Bark Side: It's a Dog's Life!

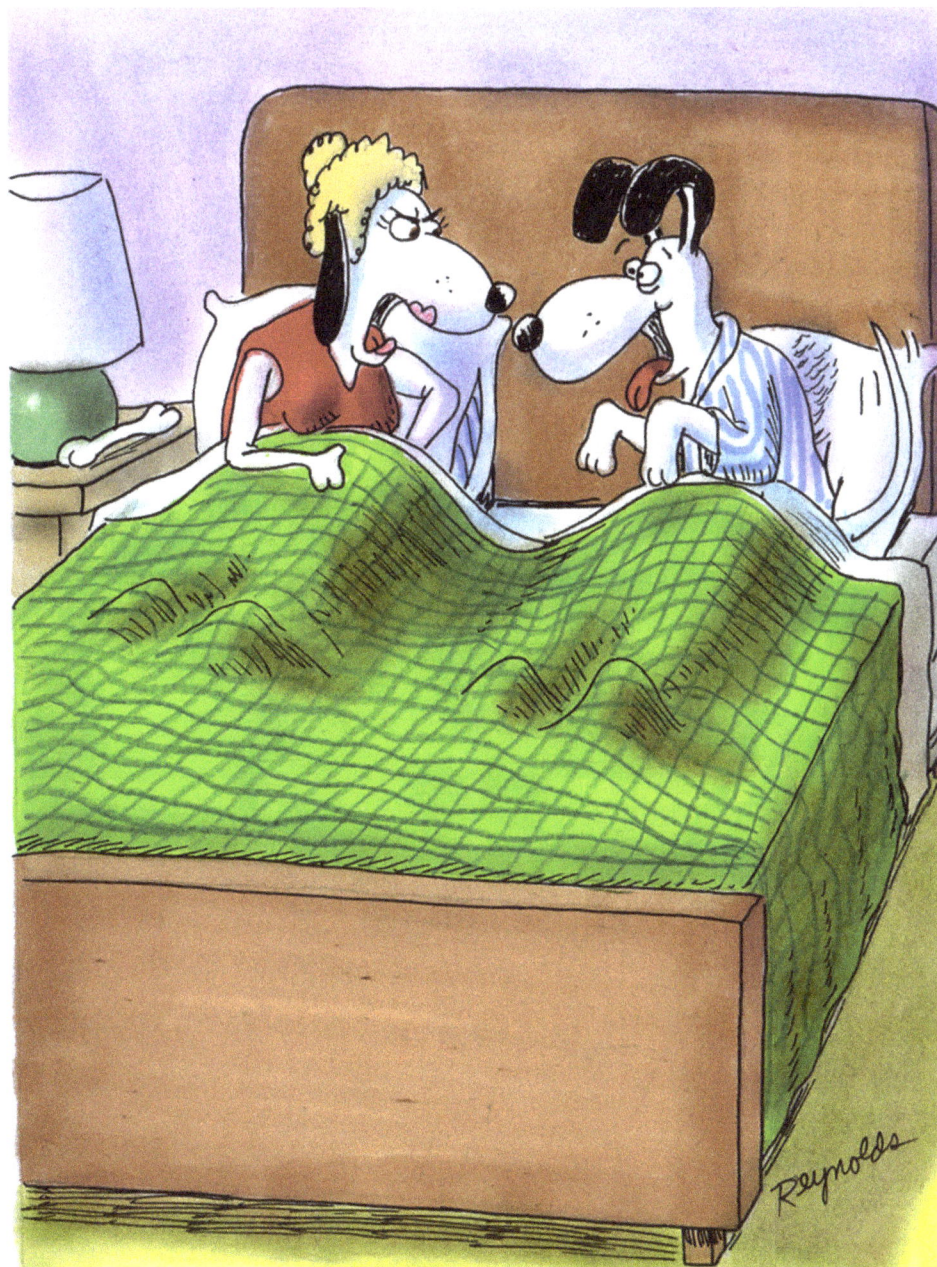

"I hate it when you beg."

The Bark Side: It's a Dog's Life!

In addition to sweating through their paw pads, dogs pant to cool themselves off. A panting dog can take 300-400 breaths (compared to his regular 30-40) with very little effort.

All dogs can be traced back 40 million years ago to a weasel-like animal called the Miacis which dwelled in trees and dens. The Miacis later evolved into the Tomarctus, a direct forbear of the genus Canis, which includes the wolf and jackal as well as the dog.

Small quantities of grapes and raisins can cause renal failure in dogs. Chocolate, macadamia nuts, cooked onions, or anything with caffeine can also be harmful.

In 2003, Dr. Roger Mugford invented the "wagometer," a device that claims to interpret a dog's exact mood by measuring the wag of its tail.

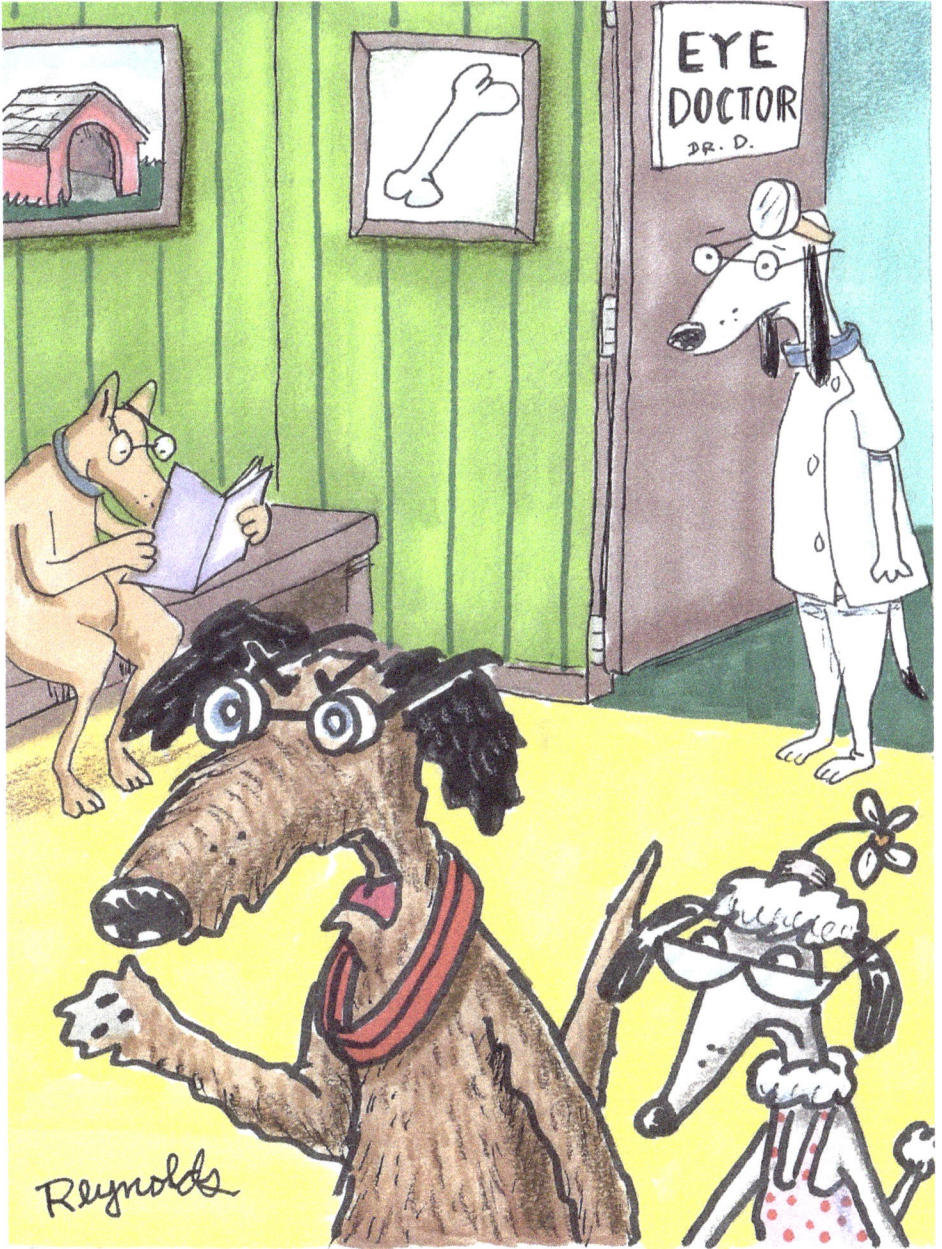

"You better believe I'm getting a second opinion... **CAT**aracts, my eye!"

The Bark Side: It's a Dog's Life!

Apple and pear seeds contain arsenic, which may be deadly to dogs.

The ancient Egyptian word for dog was "iwiw," which referred to the dog's bark

Ancient Egyptians revered their dogs. When a pet dog would die, the owners shaved off their eyebrows, smeared mud in their hair, and mourned aloud for days.

The Australian Shepherd is not actually from Australia—they are an American breed.

A dog's shoulder blades are unattached to the rest of the skeleton to allow greater flexibility for running.

Puppies are sometimes rejected by their mother if they are born by cesarean and cleaned up before being given back to her.

The Bark Side: It's a Dog's Life!

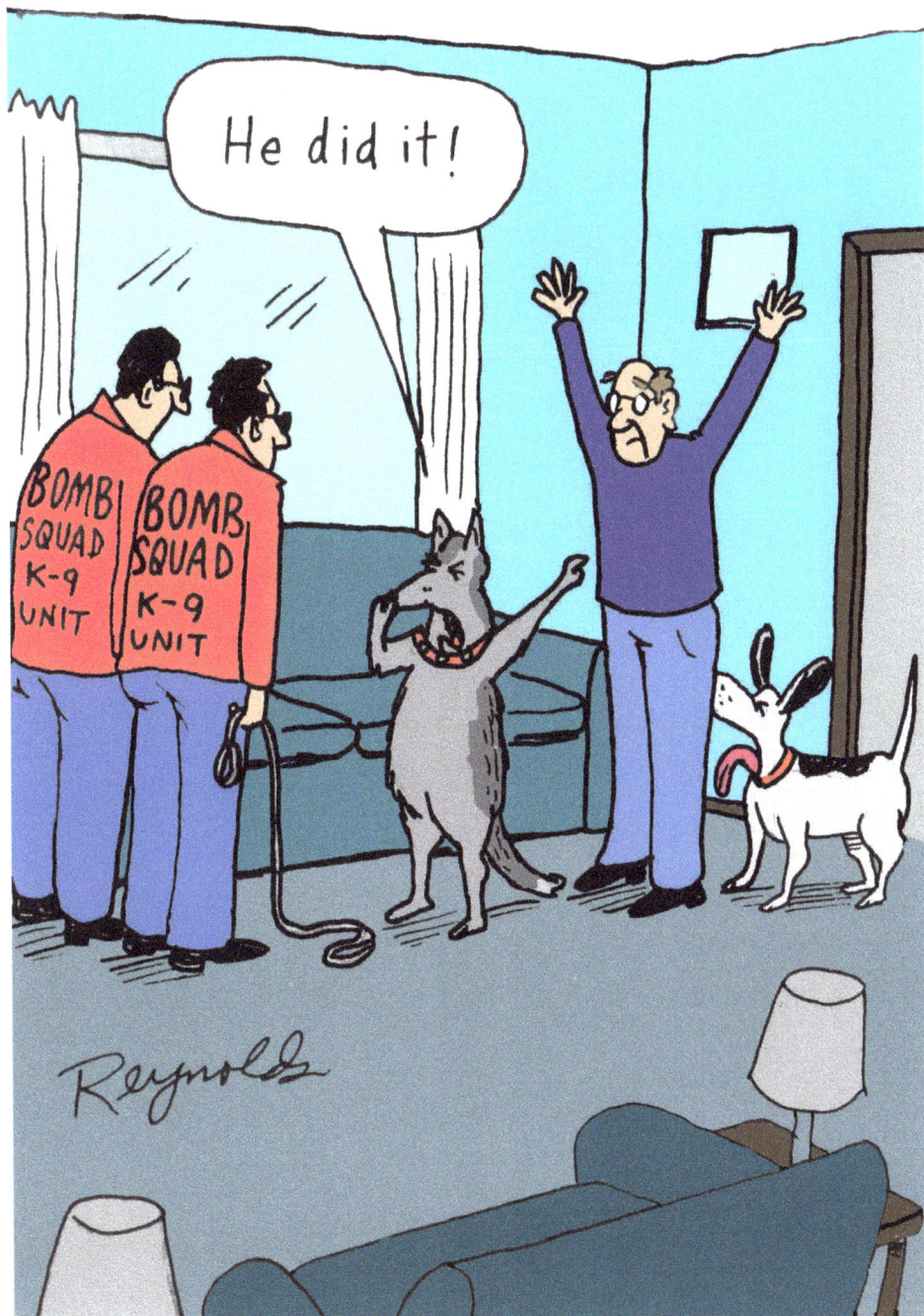

The Bark Side: It's a Dog's Life!

The phrase "raining cats and dogs" originated in seventeenth-century England. During heavy rainstorms, many homeless animals would drown and float down the streets, giving the appearance that it had actually rained cats and dogs.

During the Middle Ages, Great Danes and Mastiffs were sometimes suited with armor and spiked collars to enter a battle or to defend supply caravans.

Pekingese and Japanese Chins were so important in the ancient Far East that they had their own servants and were carried around trade routes as gifts for kings and emperors. Pekingese were even worshipped in the temples of China for centuries.

The word "werewolf" derives from Old English compound "were" (meaning "man") and "wulf" (meaning "wolf")

The Bark Side: It's a Dog's Life!

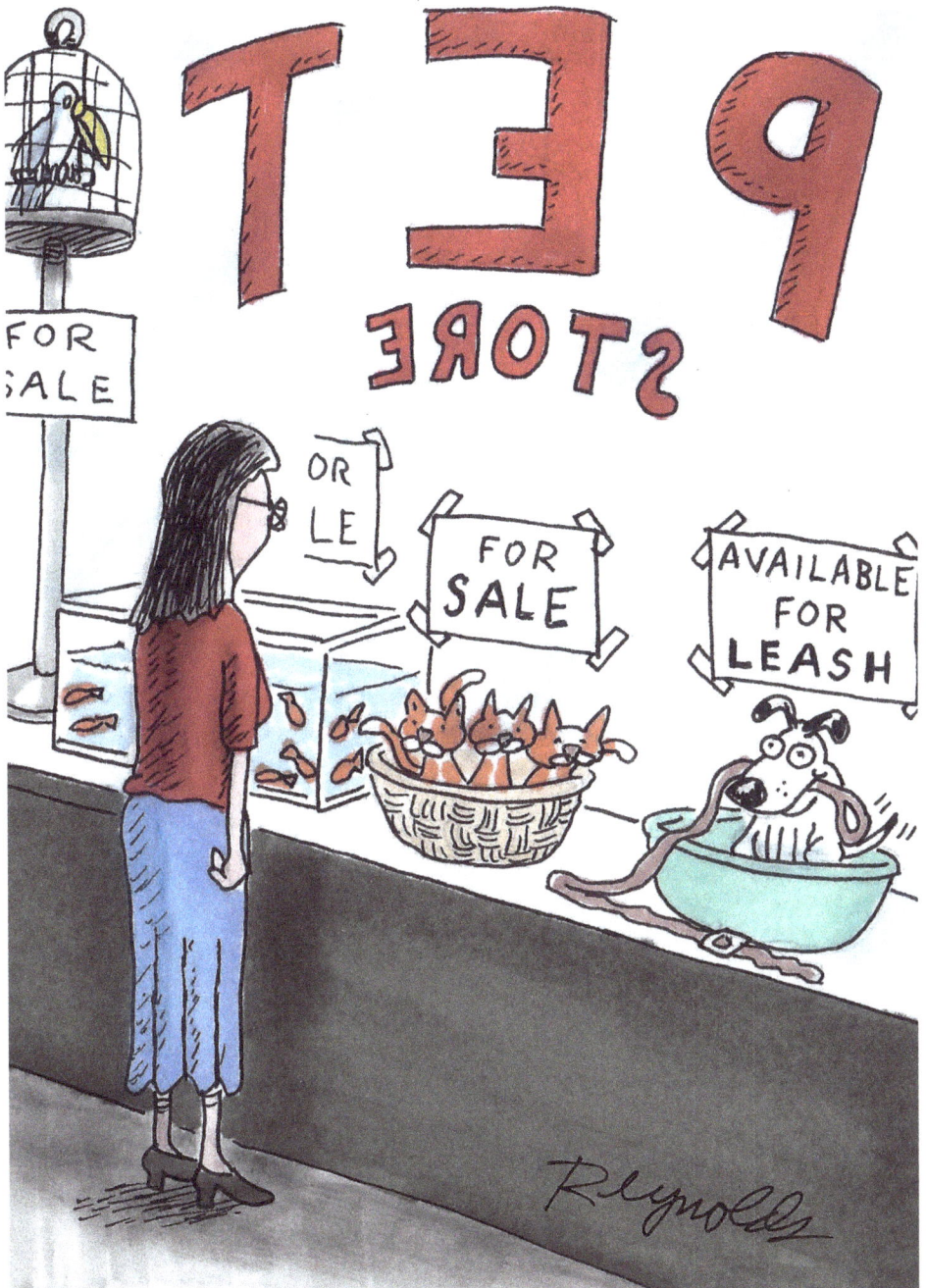

The Bark Side: It's a Dog's Life!

Dogs have sweat glands in between their paws.

After the fall of Rome, human survival often became more important than breeding and training dogs. Legends of werewolves emerged during this time as abandoned dogs traveling in packs commonly roamed streets and terrified villagers.

The American Kennel Club, the most influential dog club in the United States, was founded in 1884.

The most popular male dog names are Max and Jake. The most popular female dog names are Maggie and Molly.

Weird dog laws include allowing police offers in Palding, Ohio, to bite a dog to quiet it. In Ventura County, California, cats and dogs are not allowed to have sex without a permit.

The Bark Side: It's a Dog's Life!

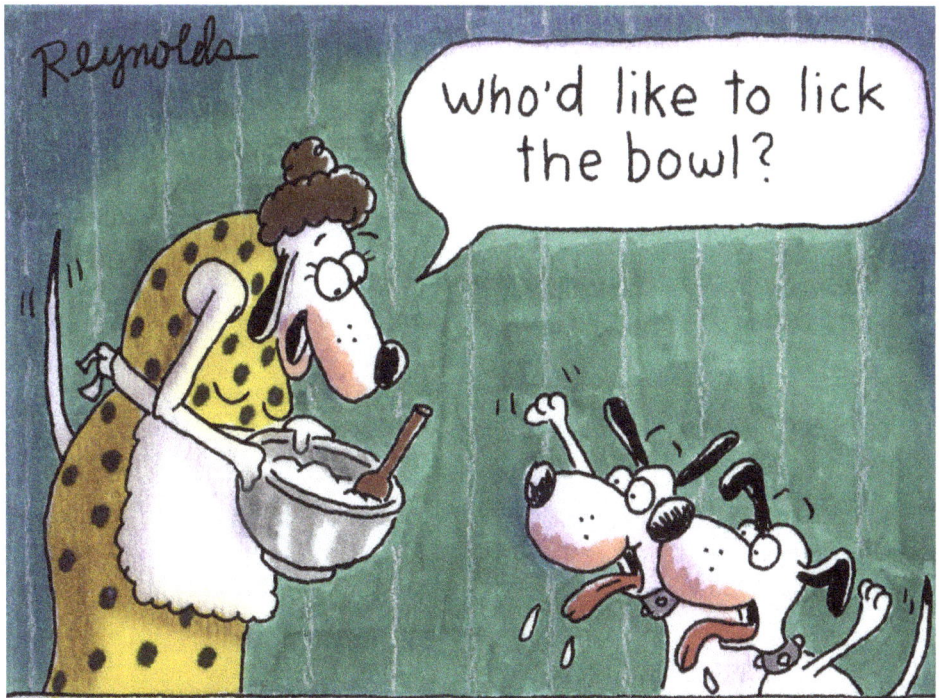

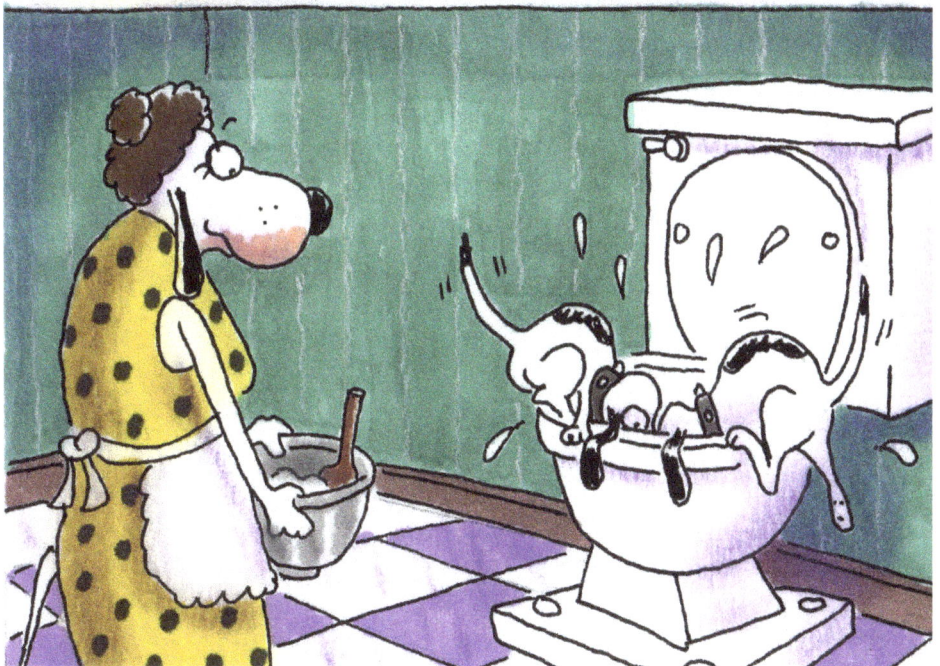

The first dog chapel was established in 2001. It was built in St. Johnsbury, Vermont, by Stephan Huneck, a children's book author whose five dogs helped him recuperate from a serious illness.

Those born under the sign of the dog in Chinese astrology are considered to be loyal and discreet, though slightly temperamental.

In Iran, it is against the law to own a dog as a pet. However, if an owner can prove the dog is a guard or hunting dog, this restriction doesn't apply. Muslim reticence concerning dogs is perhaps due to the fact that rabies has always been endemic in the Middle East.

The Mayans and Aztecs symbolized every tenth day with the dog, and those born under this sign were believed to have outstanding leadership skills.

The Bark Side: It's a Dog's Life!

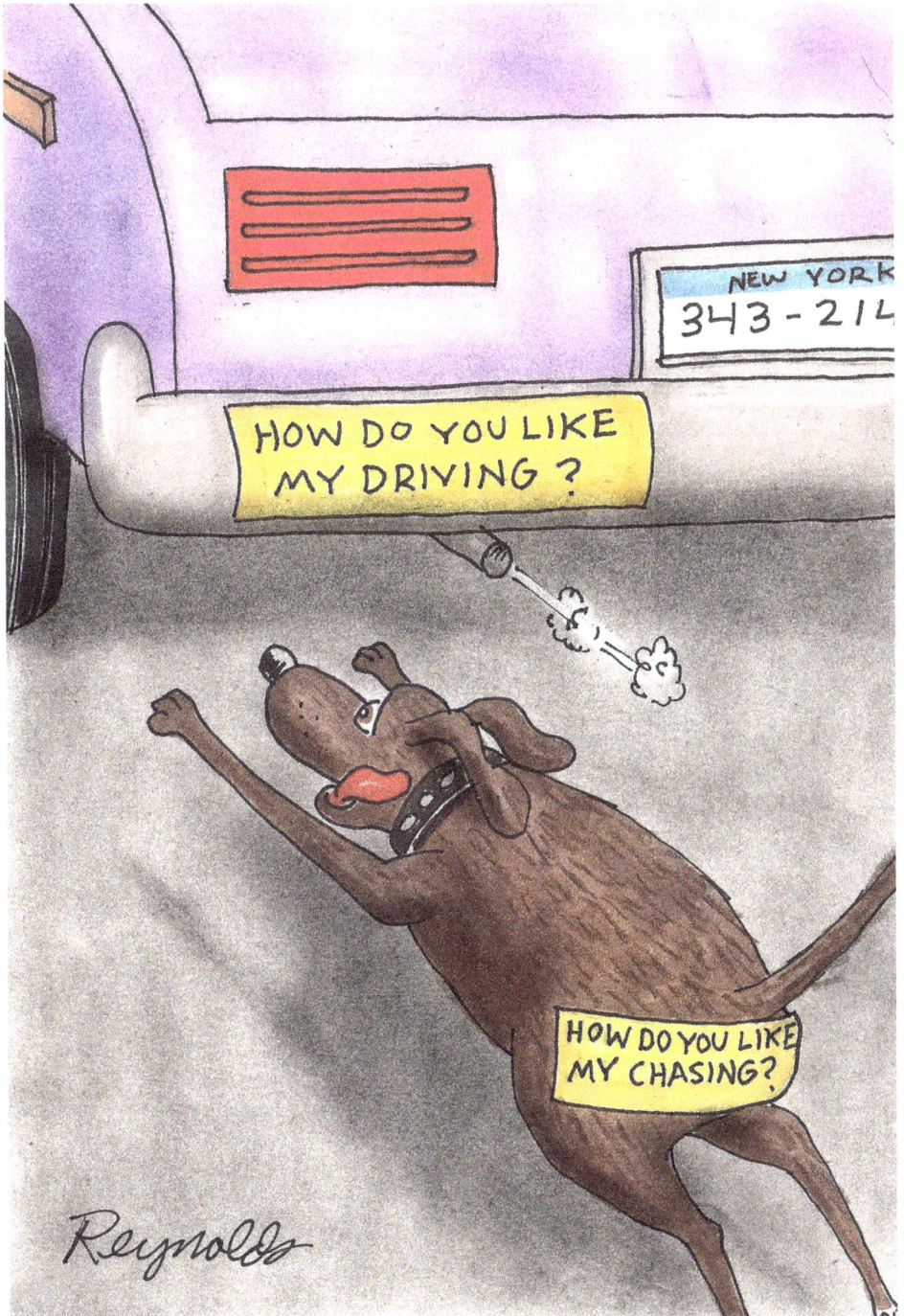

Plato once said that "a dog has the soul of a philosopher."

The most dogs ever owned by one person were 5,000 Mastiffs owned by Kublai Khan.

The shape of a dog's face suggests how long it will live. Dogs with sharp, pointed faces that look more like wolves typically live longer. Dogs with very flat faces, such as bulldogs, often have shorter lives.

French poodles did not originate in France but in Germany ("poodle" comes from the German pudel or pudelhund, meaning "splashing dog"). Some scholars speculate the poodle's puffs of hair evolved when hunters shaved the poodle for more efficient swimming, while leaving the pom-poms around the major joints to keep them warm.

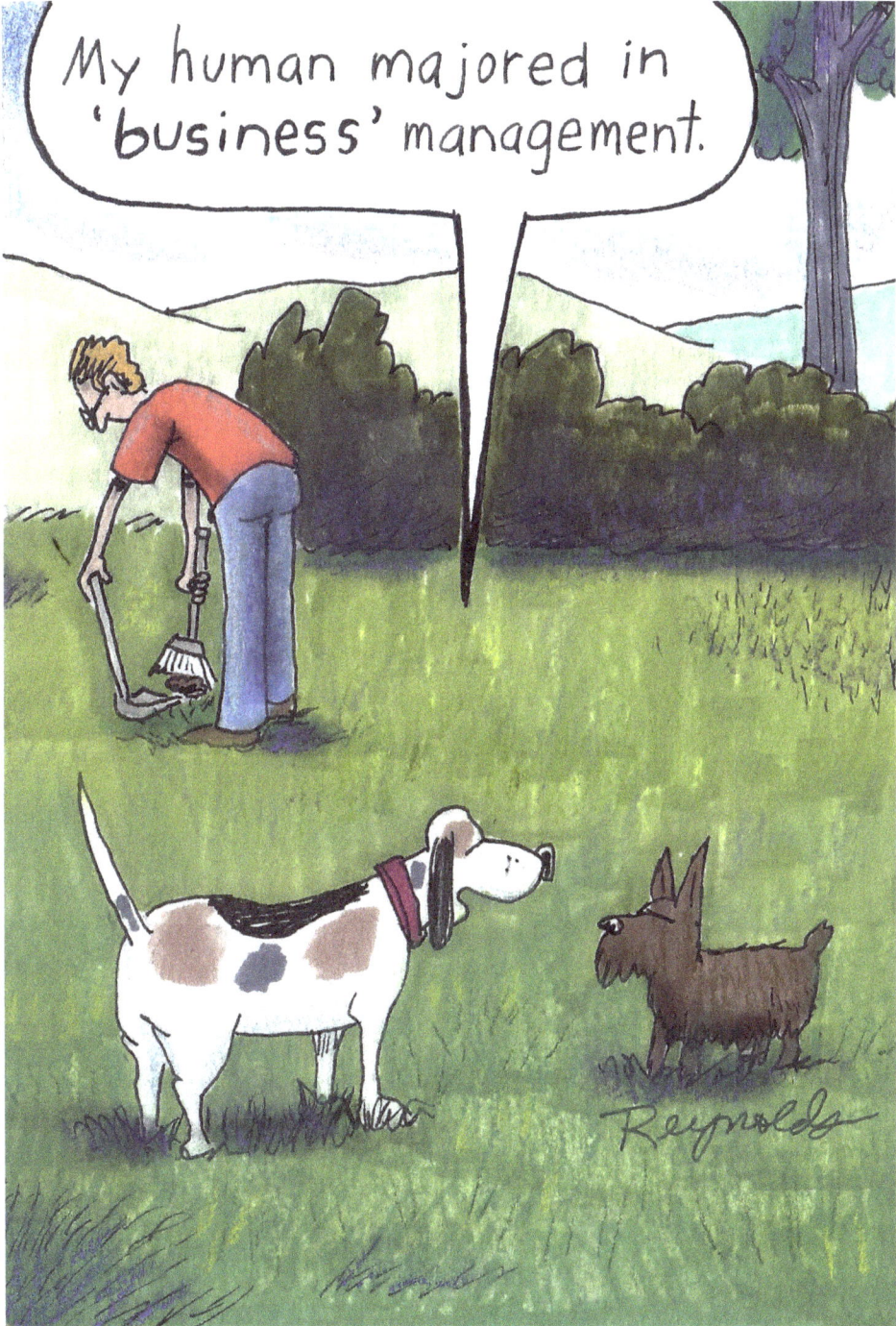

The Bark Side: It's a Dog's Life!

The ancient Mbaya Indians of the Gran Chaco in South America believed that humans originally lived underground until dogs dug them up.

The name of the dog on the Cracker Jacks box is Bingo. The Taco Bell Chihuahua is a rescued dog named Gidget.

The first dogs were self-domesticated wolves which, at least 12,000 years ago, became attracted to the first sites of permanent human habitation.

Dachshunds were bred to fight badgers in their dens.

Laika, a Russian stray, was the first living mammal to orbit the Earth, in the Soviet Sputnik spacecraft in 1957. Though she died in space, her daughter Pushnika had four puppies with President John F. Kennedy's terrier, Charlie.

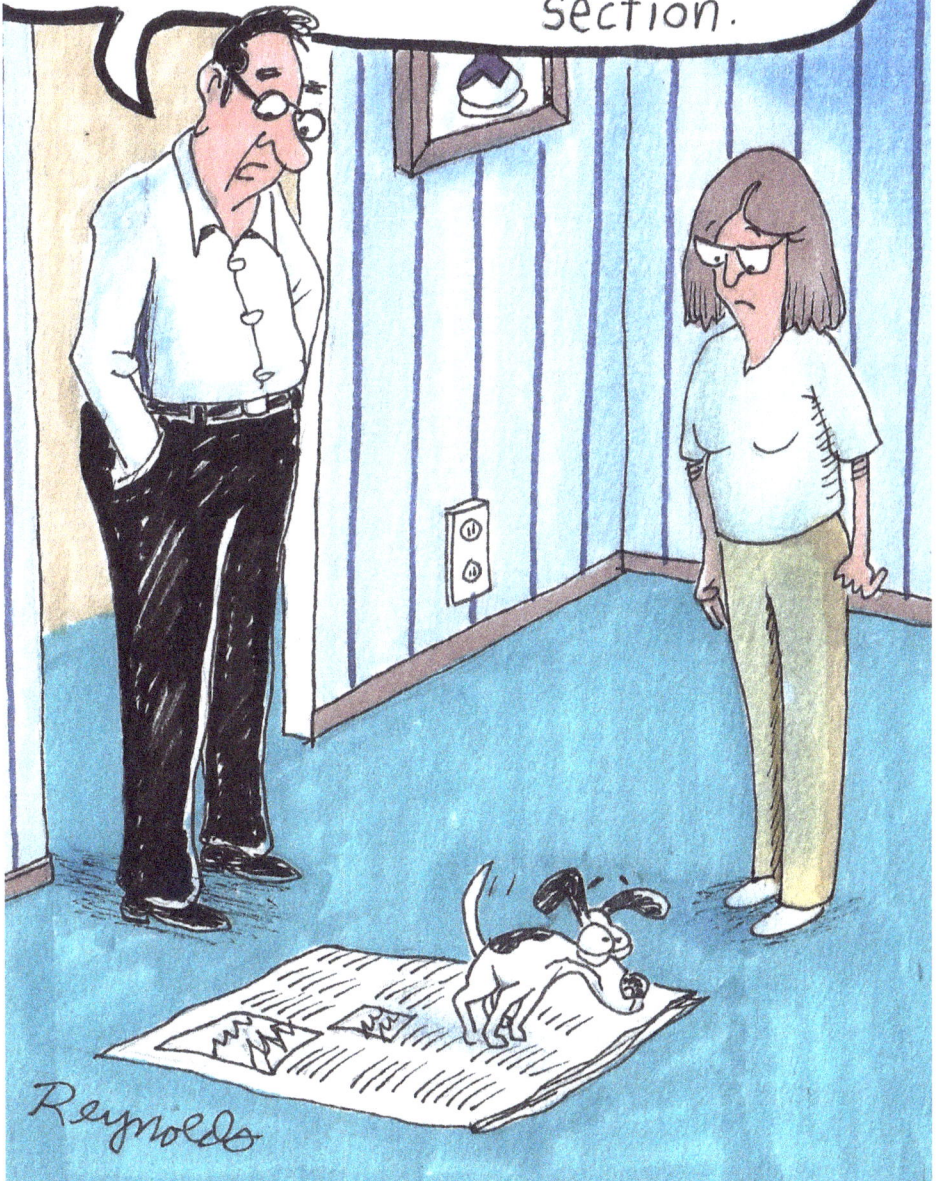

The term "dog days of summer" was coined by the ancient Greeks and Romans to describe the hottest days of summer that coincided with the rising of the Dog Star, Sirius.

In ancient Greece, kennels of dogs were kept at the sanctuary of Asclepius at Epidaurus. Dogs were frequently sacrificed there because they were plentiful, inexpensive, and easy to control. During the July 25 celebration of the *kunophontis* ("the massacre of dogs"), dog sacrifices were performed to appease the ancestors of Apollo's son, Linos, who was devoured by dogs.

Dog trainers in ancient China were held in high esteem. A great deal of dog domestication also took place in China, especially dwarfing and miniaturization.

A puppy is born blind, deaf, and toothless.

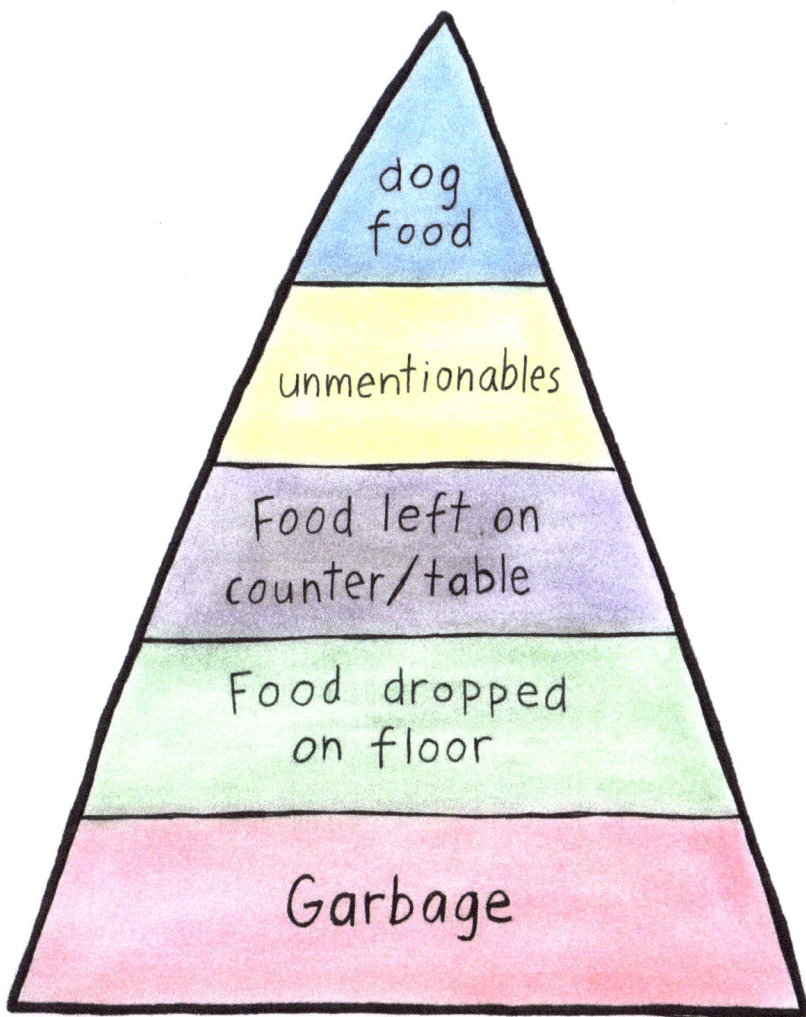

A Dog's Food Pyramid

The Bark Side: It's a Dog's Life!

The earliest European images of dogs are found in cave paintings dating back 12,000 years ago in Spain.

The ancient religion Zoroastrianism includes in its religious text titled the Zend Avesta a section devoted to the care and breeding of dogs.

Alexander the Great is said to have founded and named a city Peritas, in memory of his dog.

The dog was frequently depicted in Greek art, including Cerberus, the three-headed hound guarding the entrance to the underworld, and the hunting dogs which accompanied the virgin goddess of the chase, Diana.

A dog most likely interprets a smiling person as baring their teeth, which is an act of aggression.

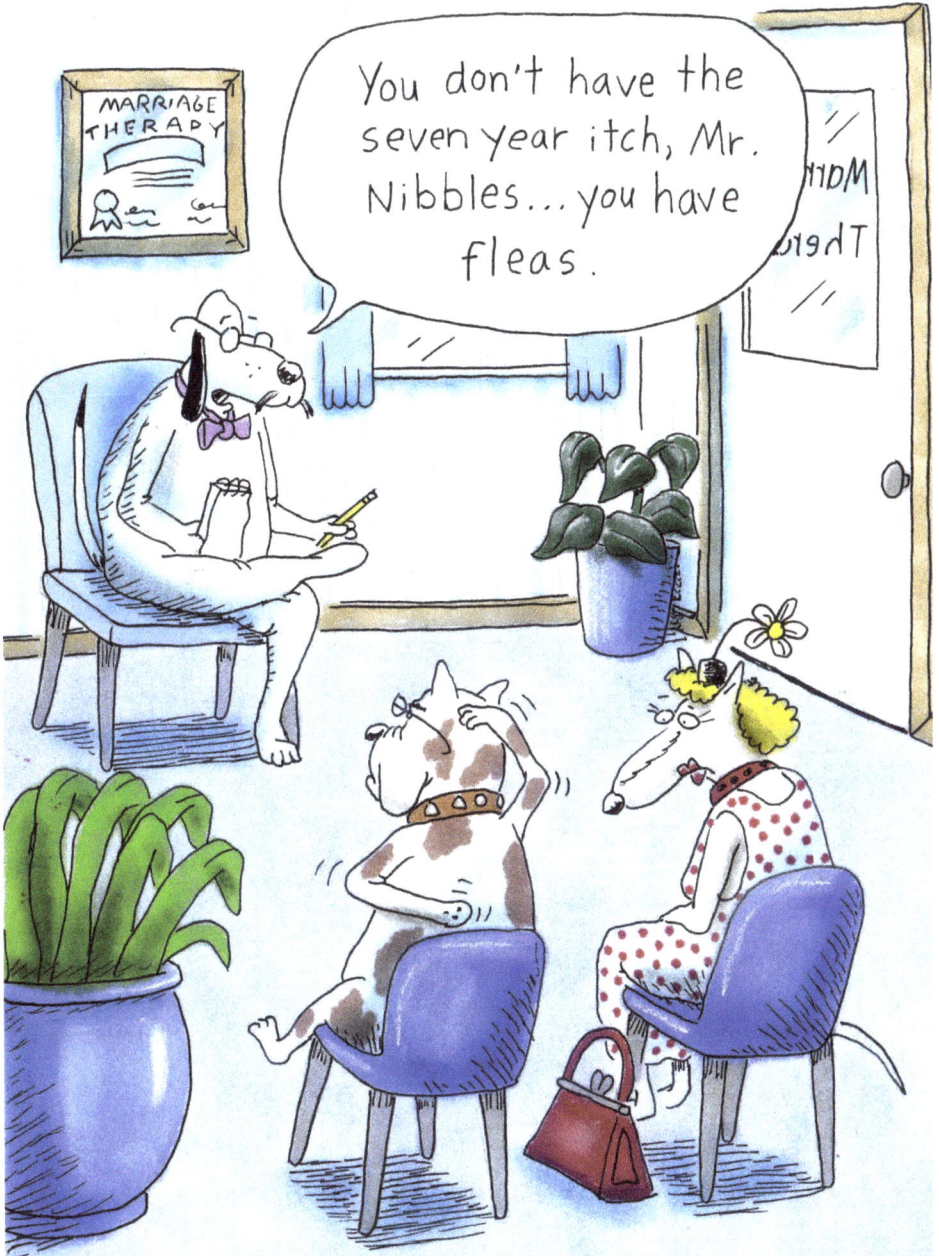

During the Renaissance, detailed portraits of the dog as a symbol of fidelity and loyalty appeared in mythological, allegorical, and religious art throughout Europe, including works by Leonardo da Vinci, Diego Velázquez, Jan van Eyck, and Albrecht Durer.

Rock star Ozzy Osborne saved his wife Sharon's Pomeranian from a coyote by tackling and wresting the coyote until it released the dog.

The origin of amputating a dog's tail may go back to the Roman writer Lucius Columella's (A.D. 4-70) assertion that tail docking prevented rabies.

One of Shakespeare's most mischievous characters is Crab, the dog belonging to Launce in the *Two Gentlemen of Verona*. The word "watchdog" is first found in *The Tempest*.

The Bark Side: It's a Dog's Life!

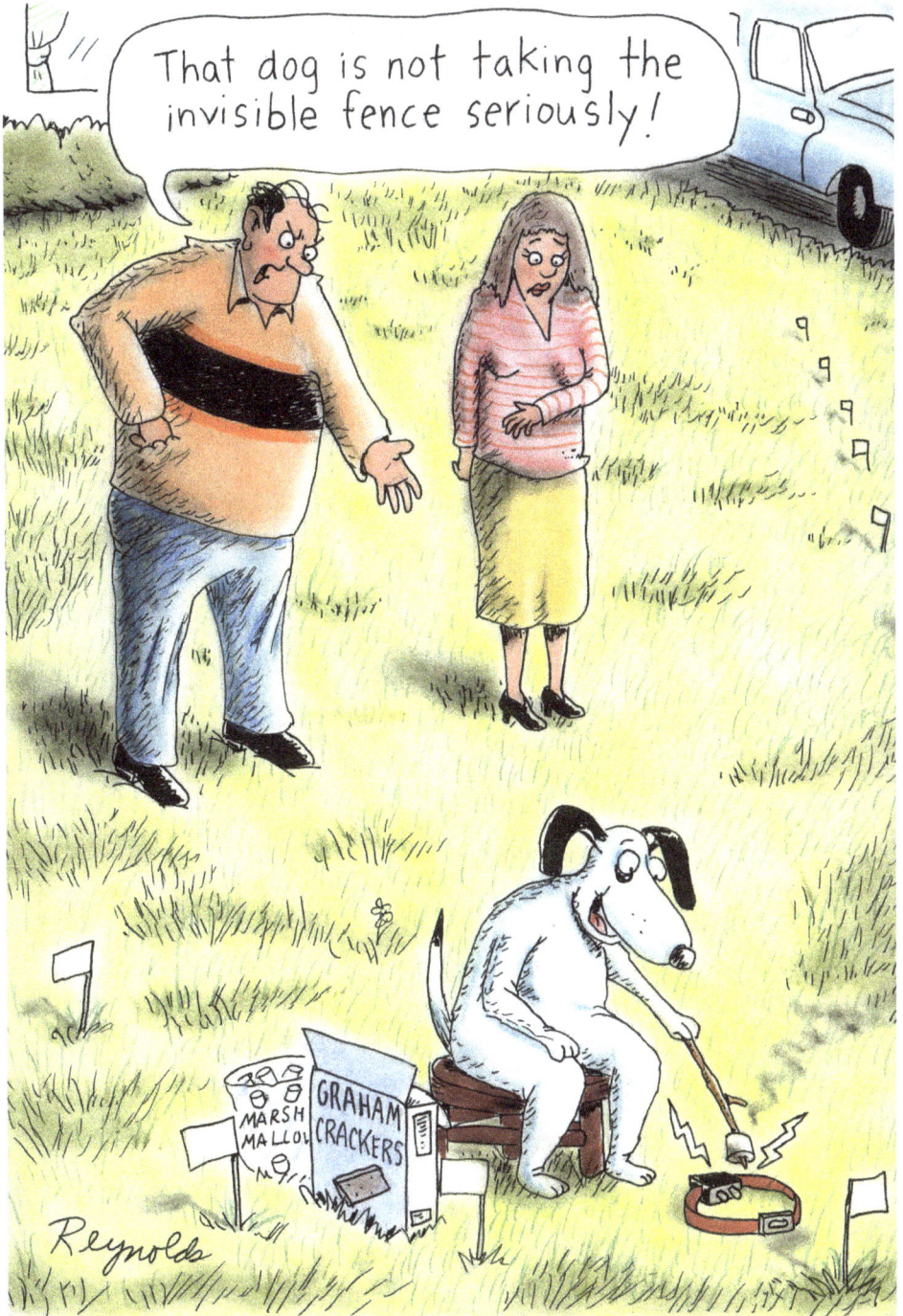

The Basenji is the world's only barkless dog.

President Franklin Roosevelt created a minor international incident when he claimed he sent a destroyer to the Aleutian Islands just to pick up his Scottish Terrier, Fala, who had been left behind.

Within hours of the September 11, 2001, attack on the World Trade Center, specially trained dogs were on the scene, including German Shepherds, Labs, and even a few little Dachshunds.

It costs approximately $10,000 to train a federally certified search and rescue dog.

The smallest dog on record was a matchbox-size Yorkshire Terrier. It was 2.5" tall at the shoulder, 3.5" from nose tip to tail, and weighed only 4 ounces.

The Bark Side: It's a Dog's Life!

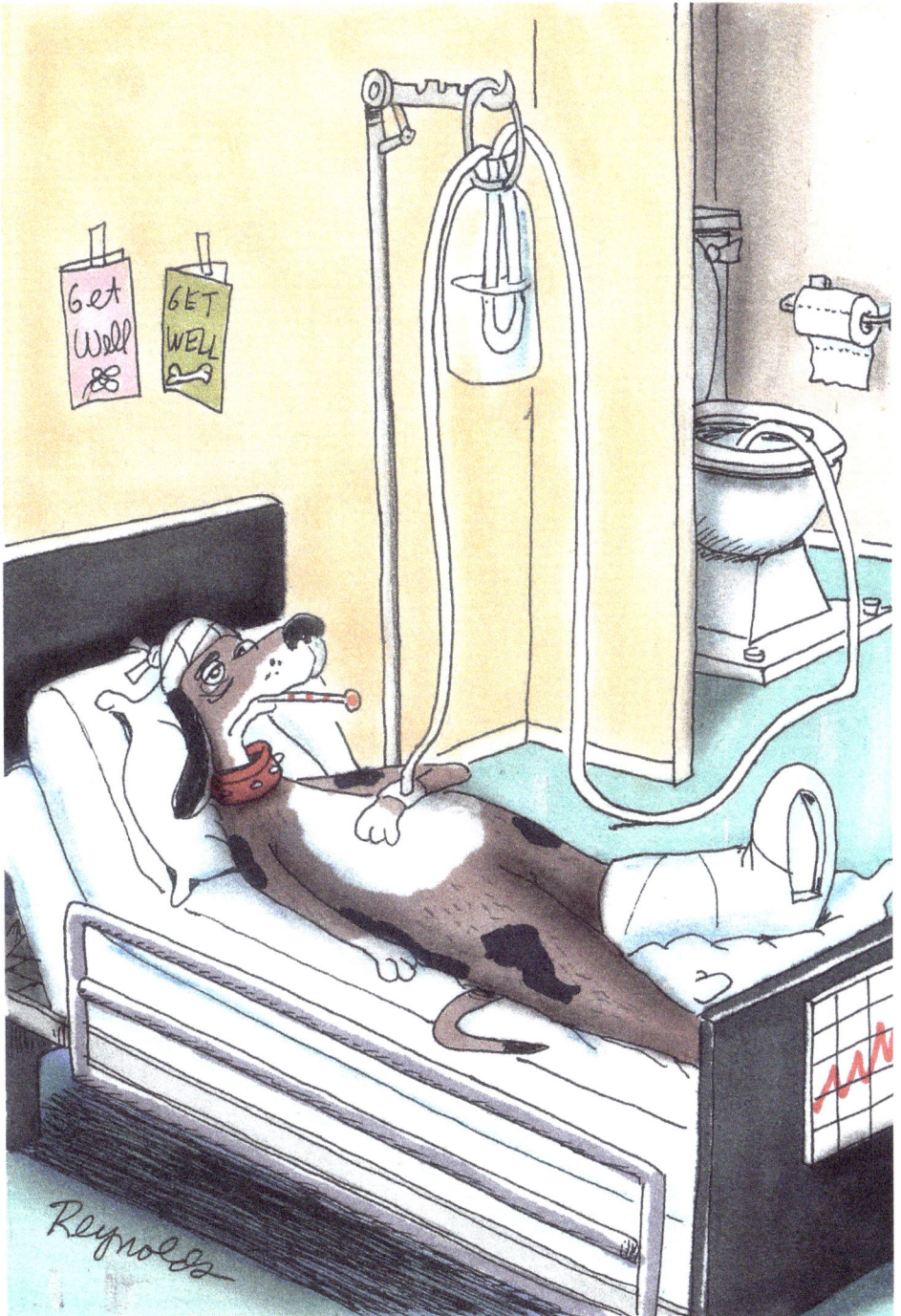

Hollywood's first and arguably best canine superstar was Rin Tin Tin, a five-day-old German Shepherd found wounded in battle in WWI France and adopted by an American soldier, Lee Duncan. He would sign his own contracts with his paw print.

In the Middle Ages, the leisured class often kept dogs as pets, while the rest of the population mainly used them for protection and herding

During the Middle Ages, mixed breeds of peasants' dogs were required to wear blocks around their necks to keep them from breeding with noble hunting dogs. Purebred dogs were very expensive and hunting became the province of the rich.

At the end of WWI, the German government trained the first guide dogs for war-blinded soldiers.

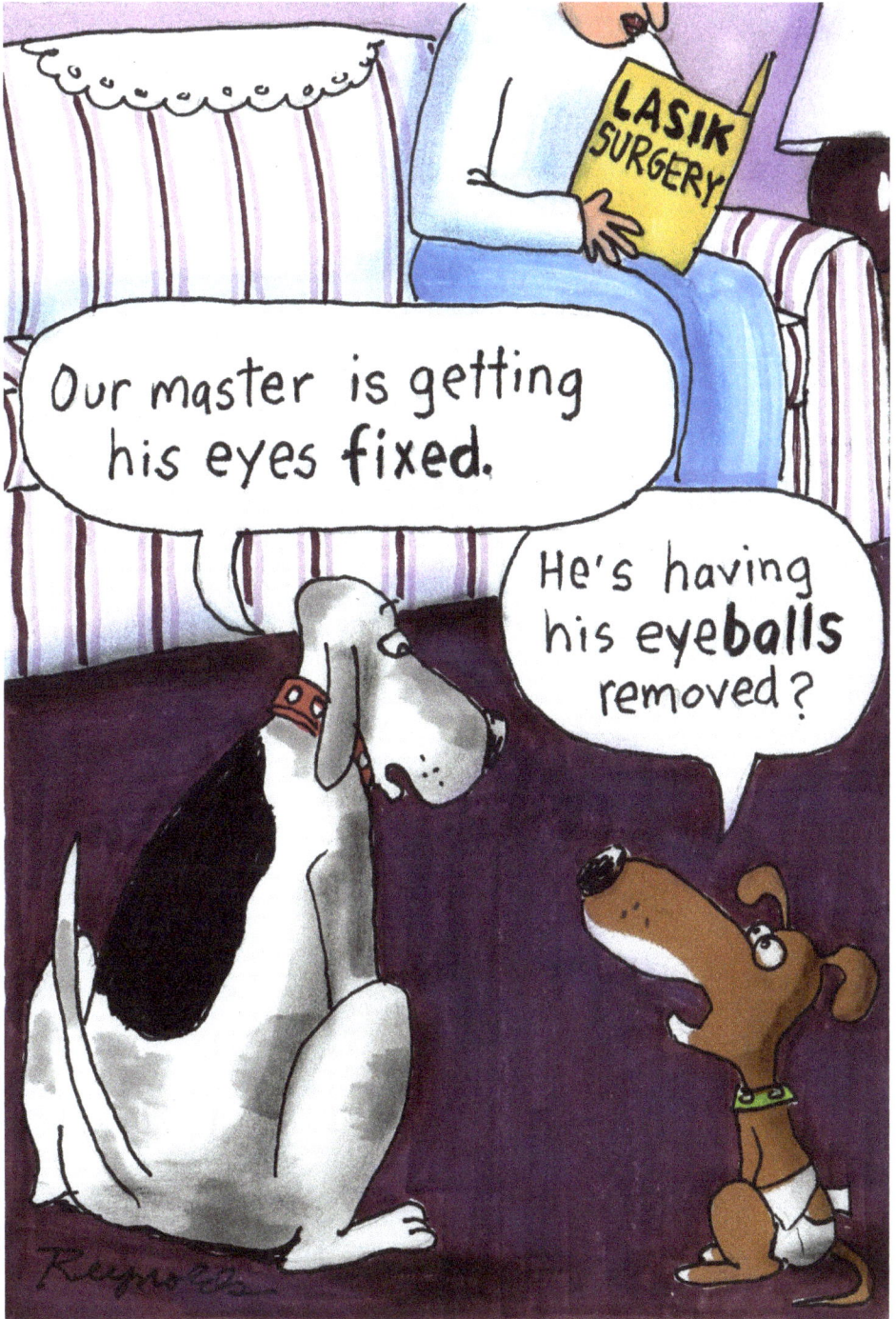

A dog can locate the source of a sound in 1/600 of a second and can hear sounds four times farther away than a human can.

Eighteen muscles or more can move a dog's ear.

The names of 77 ancient Egyptian dogs have been recorded. The names refer to color and character, such as Blackie, Ebony, Good Herdsman, Reliable, and Brave One.

In Egypt, a person bitten by a rabid dog was encouraged to eat the roasted liver of a dog infected with rabies to avoid contracting the disease. The tooth of a dog infected with rabies would also be put in a band tied to the arm of the person bitten. The menstrual blood of a female dog was used for hair removal, while dog genitals were used for preventing the whitening of hair.

The Bark Side: It's a Dog's Life!

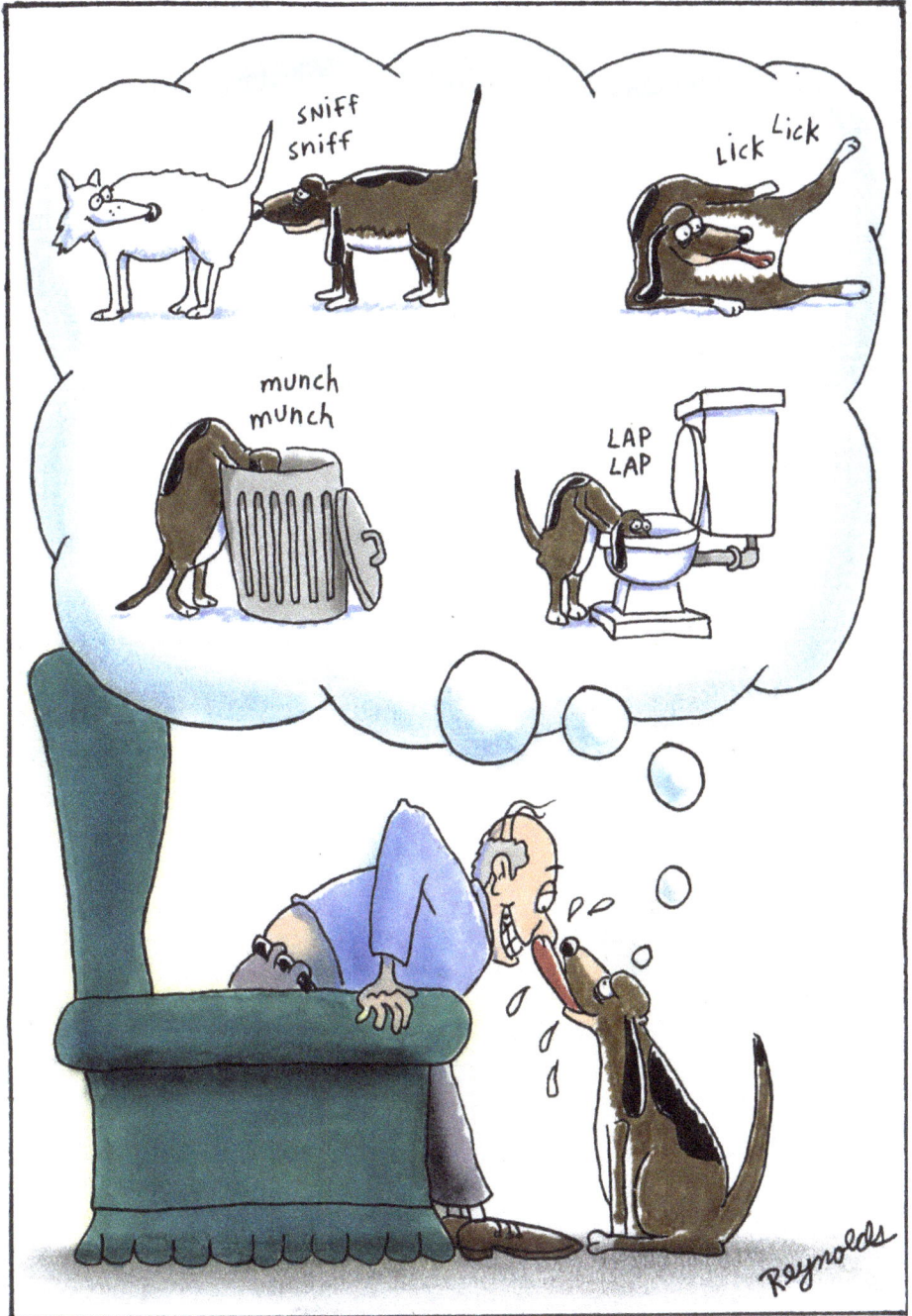

The Bark Side: It's a Dog's Life!

Touch is the first sense the dog develops. The entire body, including the paws, is covered with touch-sensitive nerve endings.

In early Christian tradition, Saint Christopher, the patron saint of travelers, is sometimes depicted with a dog's head.

The oldest known dog bones were found in Asia and date as far back as 10,000 B.C. The first identifiable dog breed appeared about 9000 B.C. and was probably a type of Greyhound dog used for hunting.

There are an estimated 400 million dogs in the world.

The U.S. has the highest dog population in the world. France has the second highest.

Toto reportedly earned $125 per week of filming, but each Munchkin actor earned just $50.

The Bark Side: It's a Dog's Life!

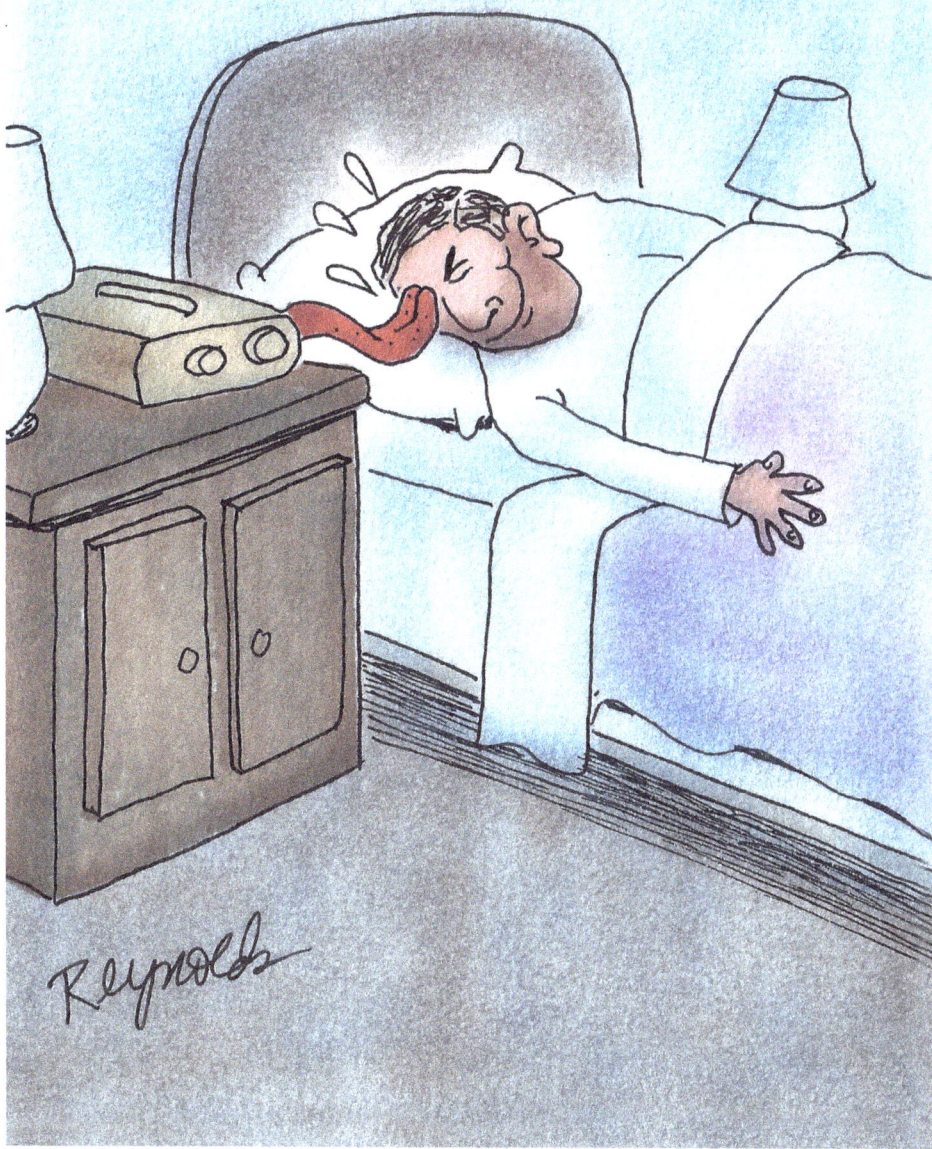

Alarm Clocks For Dog Lovers

Scholars have argued over the metaphysical interpretation of Dorothy's pooch, Toto, in the Wizard of Oz. One theory postulates that Toto represents Anubis, the dog-headed Egyptian god of death, because Toto consistently keeps Dorothy from safely returning home.

Dog nose prints are as unique as human finger prints and can be used to identify them.

Bloodhound dogs have a keen sense of smell and have been used since the Middle Ages to track criminals.

It is much easier for dogs to learn spoken commands if they are given in conjunction with hand signals or gestures.

Dogs in a pack are more likely to chase and hunt than a single dog on its own. Two dogs are enough to form a pack.

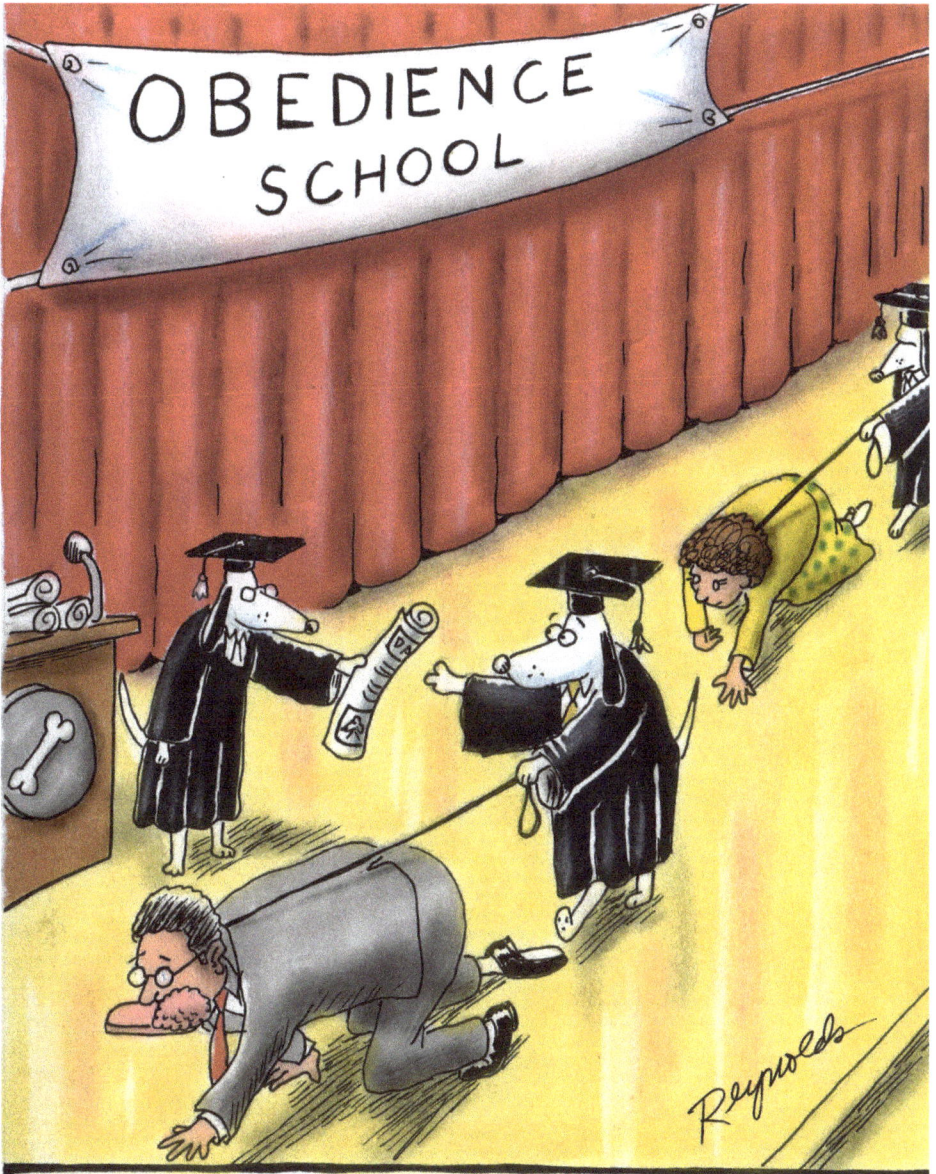

The Bark Side: It's a Dog's Life!

Dogs can see in color, though they most likely see colors similar to a color-blind human. They can see better when the light is low.

Dogs have lived with humans for over 14,000 years. Cats have lived with people for only 7,000 years.

Zorba, an English mastiff, is the biggest dog ever recorded. He weighed 343 pounds and measured 8' 3" from his nose to his tail.

The average dog can run about 19 mph. Greyhounds are the fastest dogs on Earth and can run at speeds of 45 mph.

One female dog and her female children could produce 4,372 puppies in seven years.

Petting dogs is proven to lower blood pressure of dog owners.

The Bark Side: It's a Dog's Life!

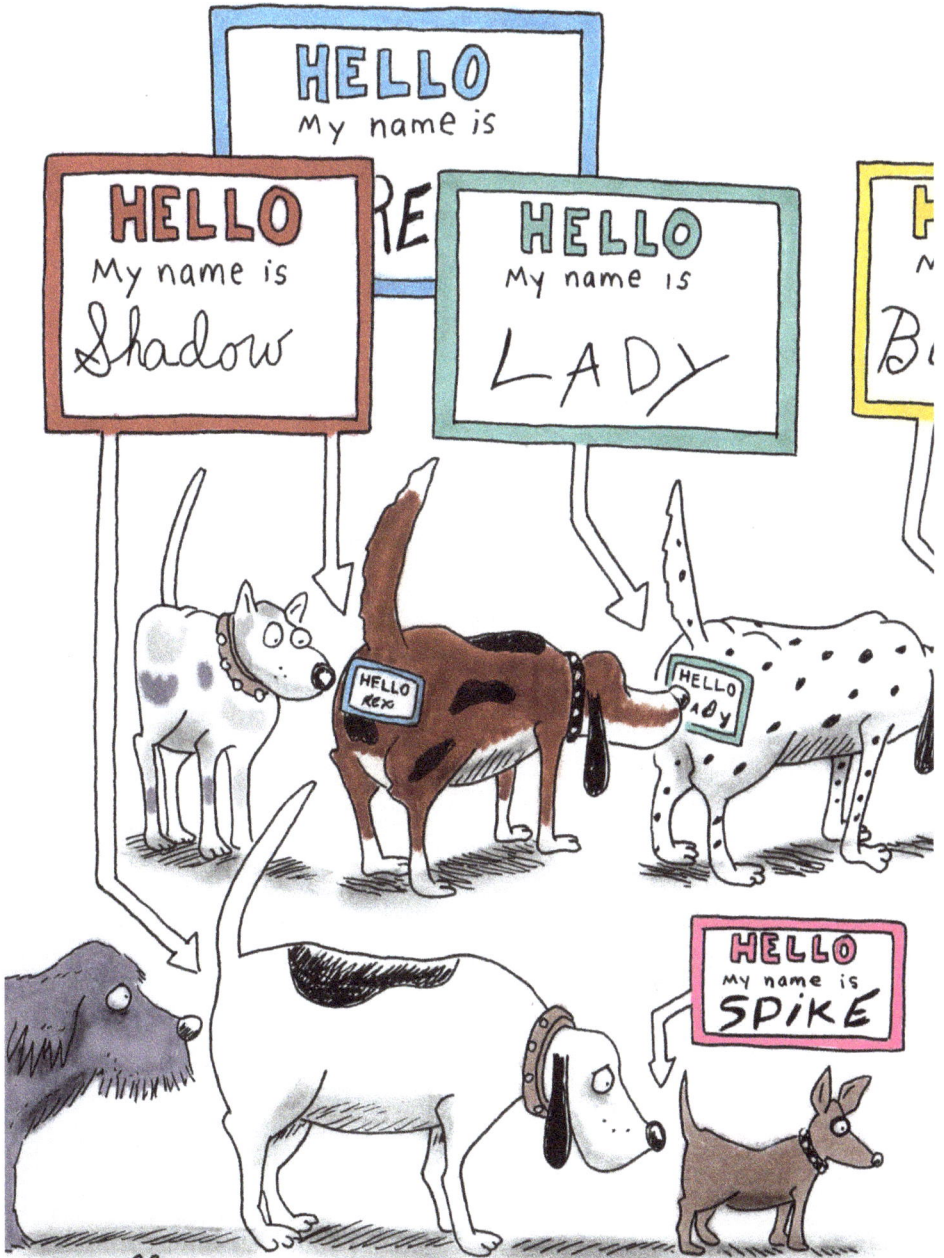

The most popular dog breed in Canada, U.S., and Great Britain is the Labrador retriever.

Greyhounds appear to be the most ancient dog breed. "Greyhound" comes from a mistake in translating the early German name Greishund, which means "old (or ancient) dog," not from the color gray.

The oldest dog on record was an Australian cattle dog named Bluey who lived 29 years and 5 months. In human years, that is more than 160 years old.

Most experts believe humans domesticated dogs before donkeys, horses, sheep, goats, cattle, cats, or chickens.

Dogs with big, square heads and large ears (like the Saint Bernard) are the best at hearing subsonic sounds.

The Bark Side: It's a Dog's Life!

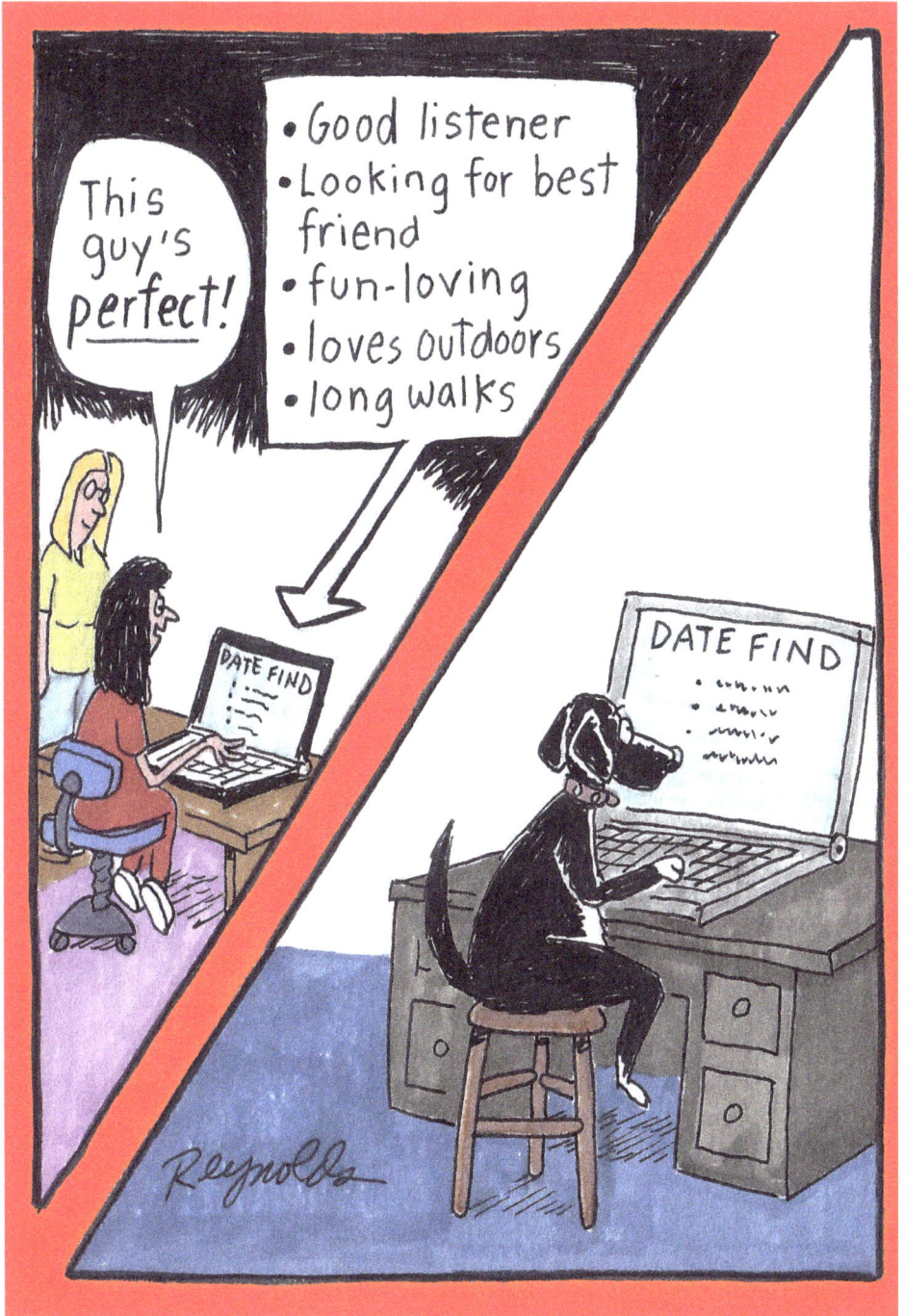

The Bark Side: It's a Dog's Life!

A person standing still 300 yards away is almost invisible to a dog. But a dog can easily identify its owner standing a mile away if the owner is waving his arms.

In Croatia, scientists discovered that lampposts were falling down because a chemical in the urine of male dogs was rotting the metal.

Dogs can smell about 1,000-10,000 times better than humans. While humans have 5 million smell-detecting cells, dogs have more than 220 million. The part of the brain that interprets smell is also four times larger in dogs than in humans.

Some dogs can smell dead bodies under water, where termites are hiding, and natural gas buried under 40 feet of dirt. They can even detect cancer that is too small to be detected by a doctor and can find lung cancer by sniffing a person's breath.

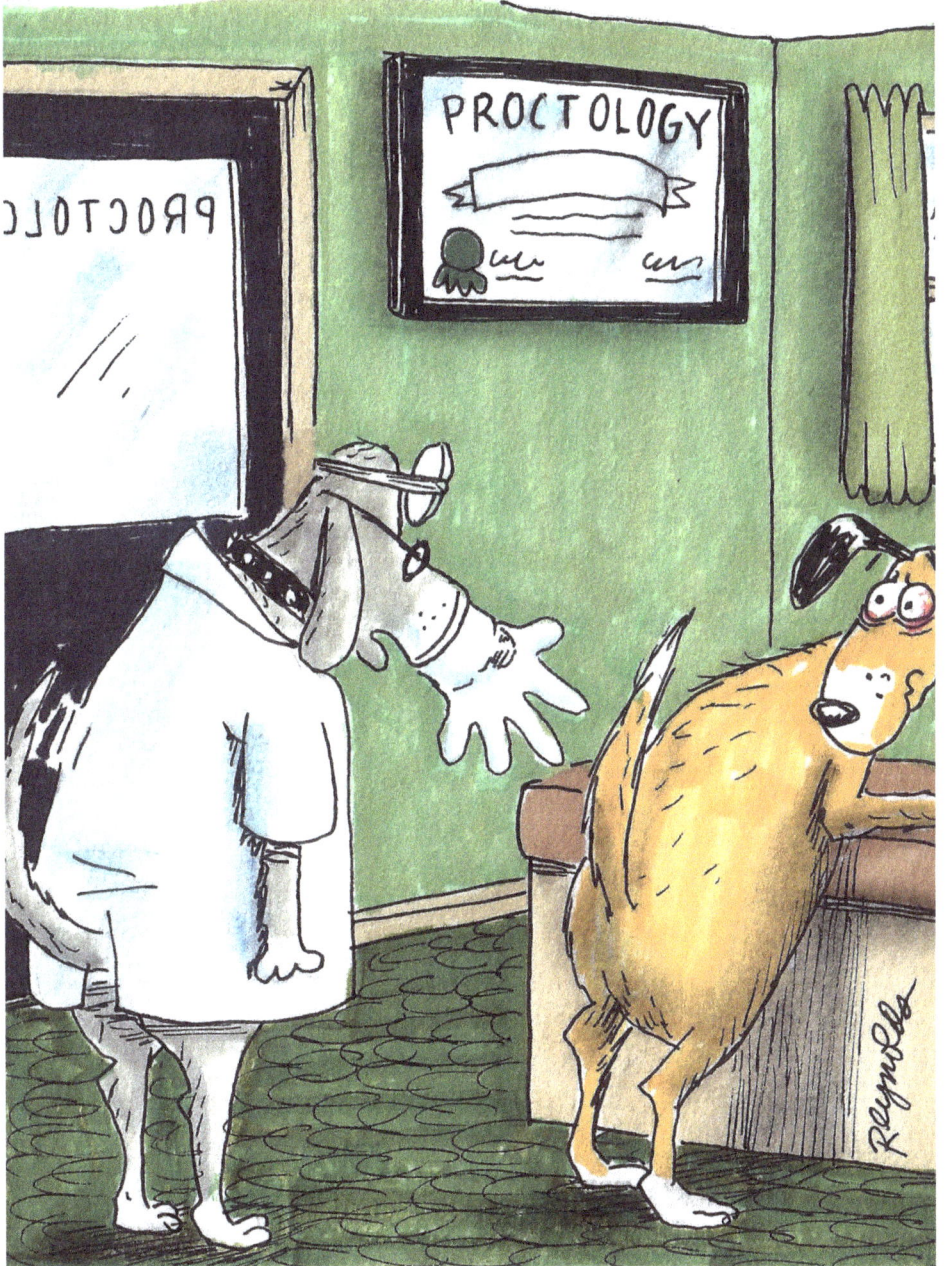

"Try to relax..."

The Bark Side: It's a Dog's Life!

Dogs have a wet nose to collect more of the tiny droplets of smelling chemicals in the air.

Dogs like sweets a lot more than cats do. While cats have around only 473 taste buds, dogs have about 1,700 taste buds. Humans have approximately 9,000.

Different smells in a dog's urine can tell other dogs whether the dog leaving the message is female or male, old or young, sick or healthy, happy or angry.

Male dogs will raise their legs while urinating to aim higher on a tree or lamppost because they want to leave a message that they are tall and intimidating. Some wild dogs in Africa try to run up tree trunks while they are urinating to appear to be very large.

Almost 1 in 5 people bitten by dogs require medical attention

The Real Reason Dogs Stick Their Heads Out of Car Windows ...

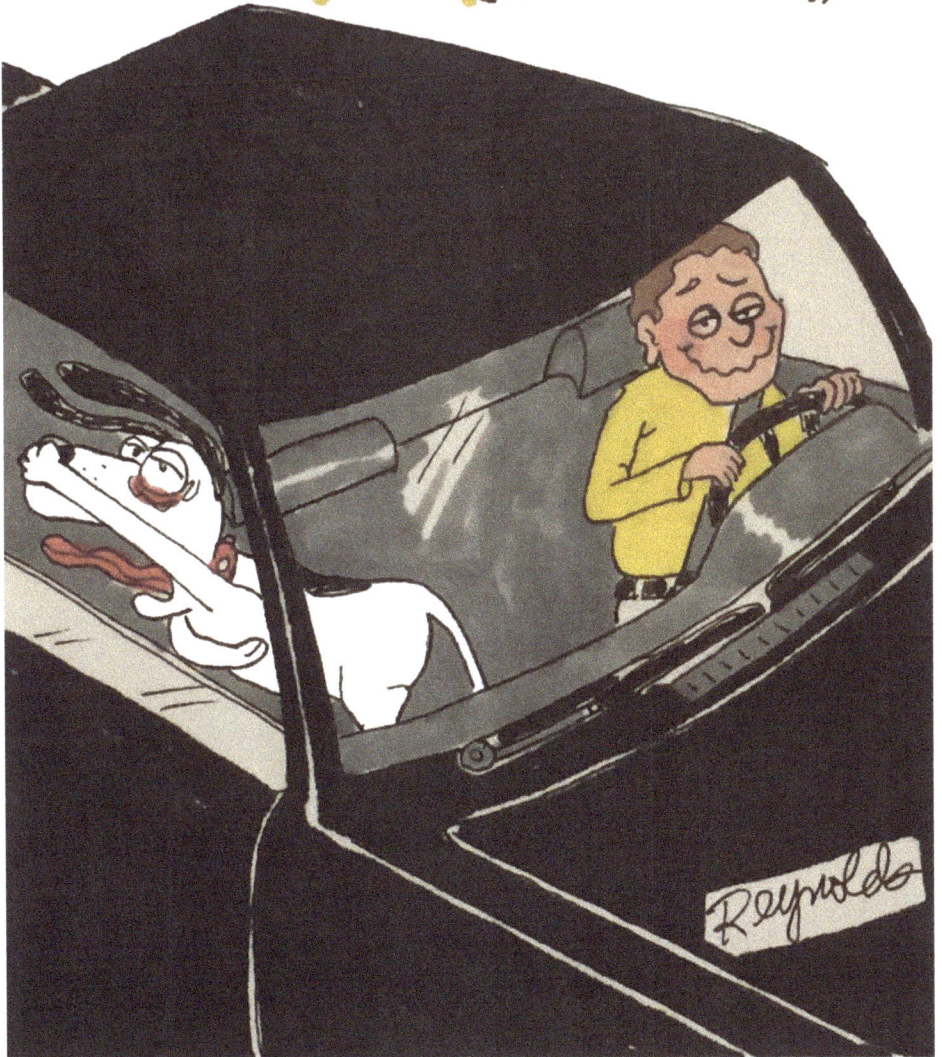

The Bark Side: It's a Dog's Life!

A lost Dachshund was found swallowed whole in the stomach of a giant catfish in Berlin on July 2003.

Countess Karlotta Libenstein of Germany left approximately $106 million to her Alsatian, Gunther III, when she died in 1992.

A person should never kick a dog facing him or her. Some dogs can bite 10 times before a human can respond.

In Australia, a man who was arrested for drug possession argued his civil rights were violated when the drug-sniffing dog nuzzled his crotch. While the judge dismissed the charges, they were later reinstated when a prosecutor pointed out that in the animal kingdom, crotch nuzzling was a friendly gesture.

A group of pugs is called a "grumble."

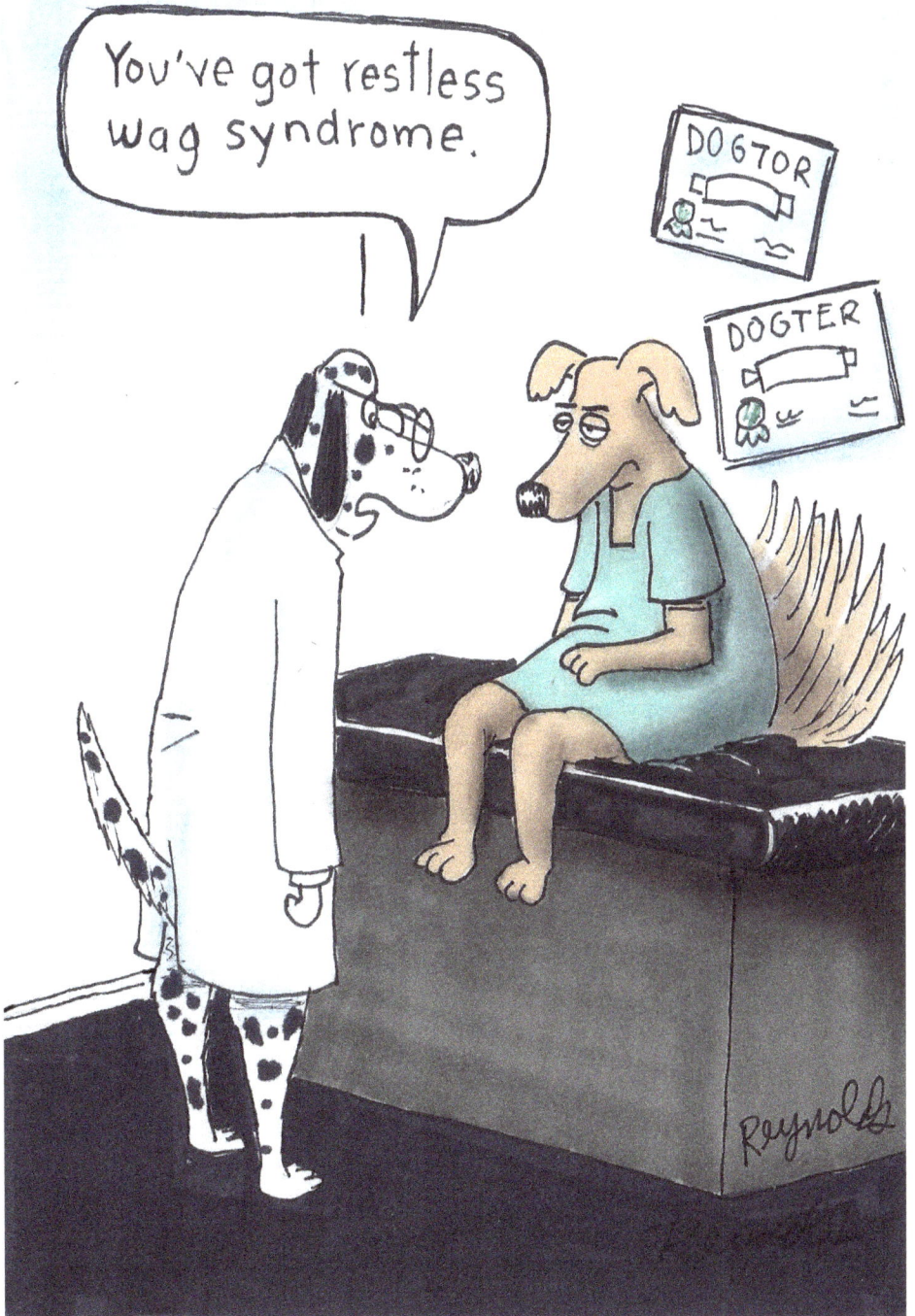

The best dog to reportedly attract a date is the Golden Retriever. The worst is the Pit Bull.

The Beagle came into prominence in the 1300s and 1400s during the days of King Henry VII of England. Elizabeth I was fond of Pocket Beagles, which were only 9" high.

The Akita is one of the most challenging dogs to own. Some insurance companies have even characterized it as the #1 "bad dog" and may even raise an Akita owner's homeowner insurance costs.

The Beagle and Collie are the nosiest dogs, while the Akbash Dog and the Basenji are the quietest.

One survey reports that 33% of dog owners admit they talk to their dogs on the phone or leave messages on answering machines while they are away.

The Bark Side: It's a Dog's Life!

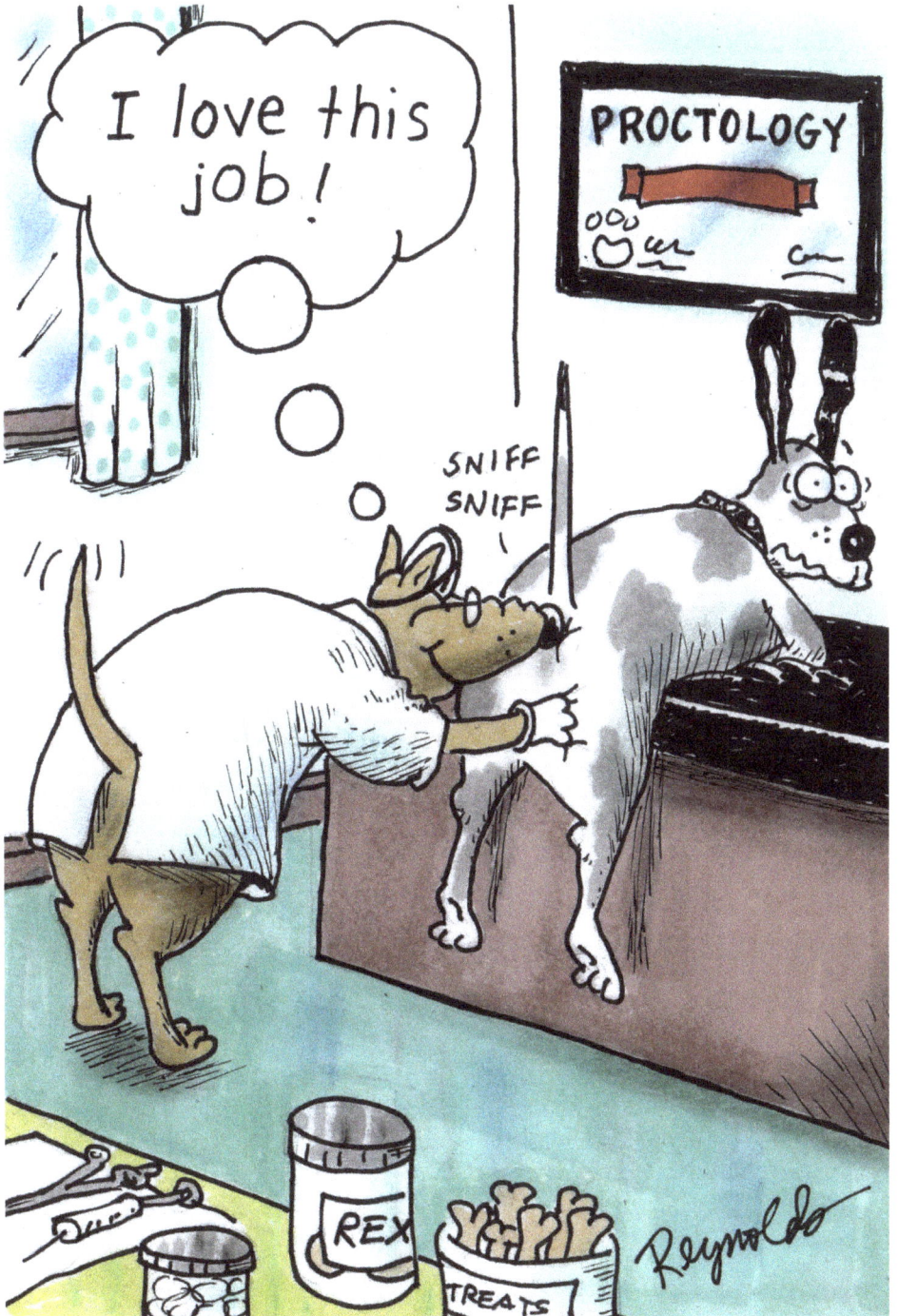

Corgi is Welsh for 'dwarf dog'.

Thirty percent of all Dalmatians are deaf in one or both ears. Because bulldogs have extremely short muzzles, many spend their lives fighting suffocation. Because Chihuahuas have such small skulls, the flow of spinal fluid can be restricted, causing hydrocephalus, a swelling of the brain.

Dogs are about as smart as a two- or three-year-old child. This means they can understand about 150-200 words, including signals and hand movements with the same meaning as words.

The grief suffered after a pet dog dies can be the same as that experienced after the death of a person.

There are almost 5 million dog bites per year; children are the main victims. Dog bites cause losses of over $1 billion a year.

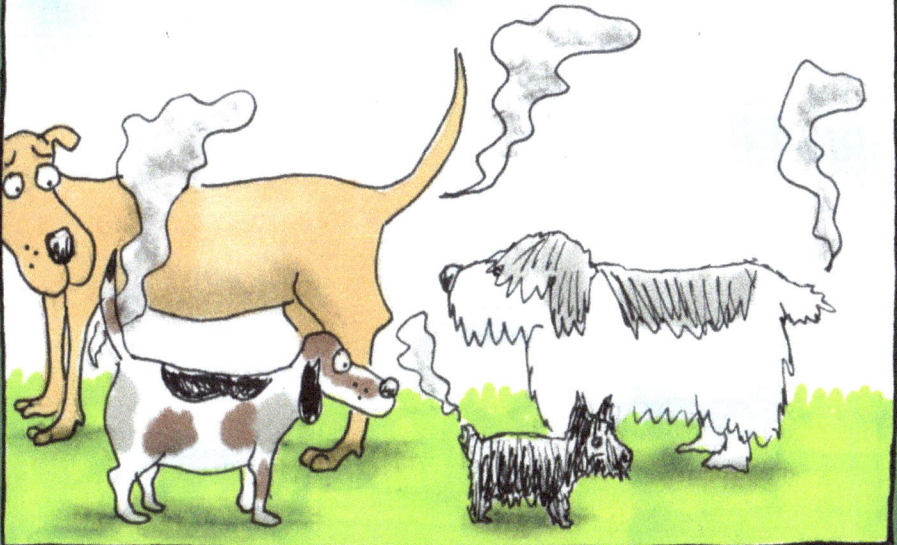

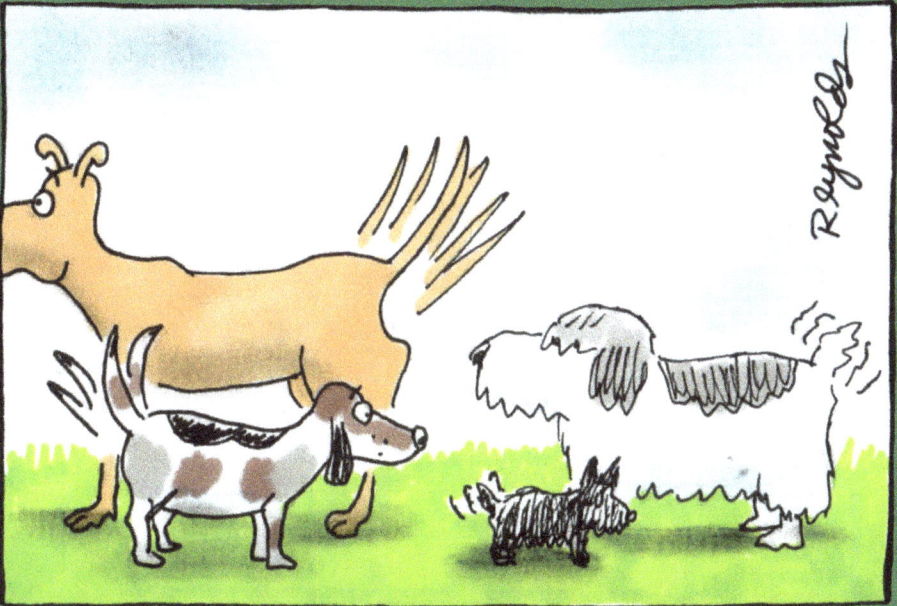

The most intelligent dogs are reportedly the Border Collie and the Poodle, while the least intelligent dogs are the Afghan Hound and the Basenji.

One kind of Pekingese is referred to as a "sleeve" because it was bred to fit into a Chinese empress' sleeves, which was how it was often carried around.

The Basenji is the only breed of dog that cannot bark, but it can yodel.

When dogs poop, they prefer to do it in alignment with the Earth's magnetic field.

If a guy has a dog with him, he is three times as likely to get a girl's phone number.

If you leave a dog a piece of clothing with your aroma it can comfort them and reduce separation anxiety.

The Bark Side: It's a Dog's Life!

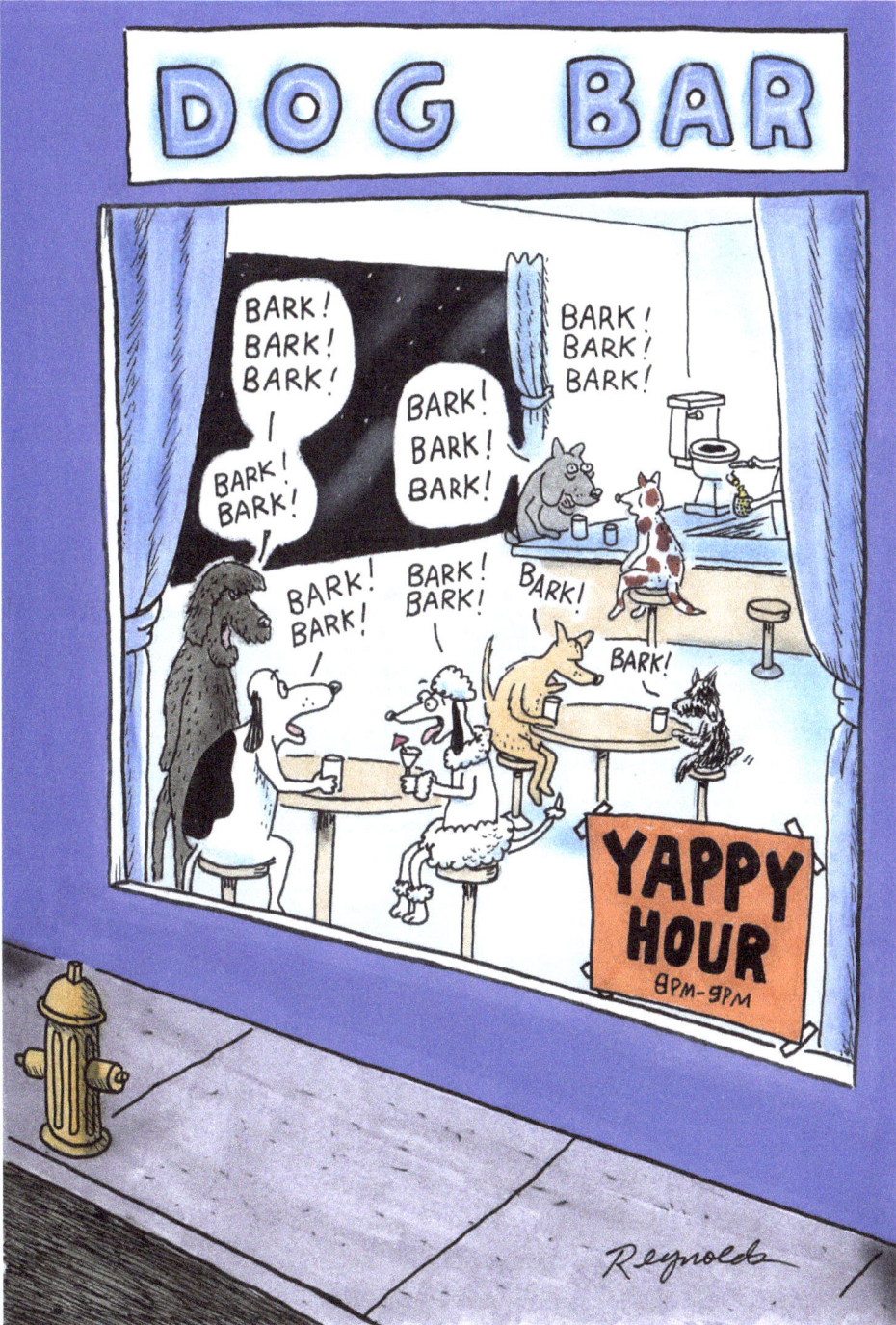

The Bark Side: It's a Dog's Life!

There are hundreds of different breeds of dogs, and around 400 million dogs in the world.

The most popular breed of dog is the Labrador, with their gentle nature, intelligence and obedience they make for excellent pets and reliable workers. They often work as guide dogs.

Dogs have much better smell than humans, and can detect different odors of nearly 100 million times lower potency than humans can.

Dogs hearing is also much better, and they can hear sounds four times further away than humans.

An average dog will live to between 10 and 14 years of age.

There are 18 different muscles that dogs use to move each one of their ears.

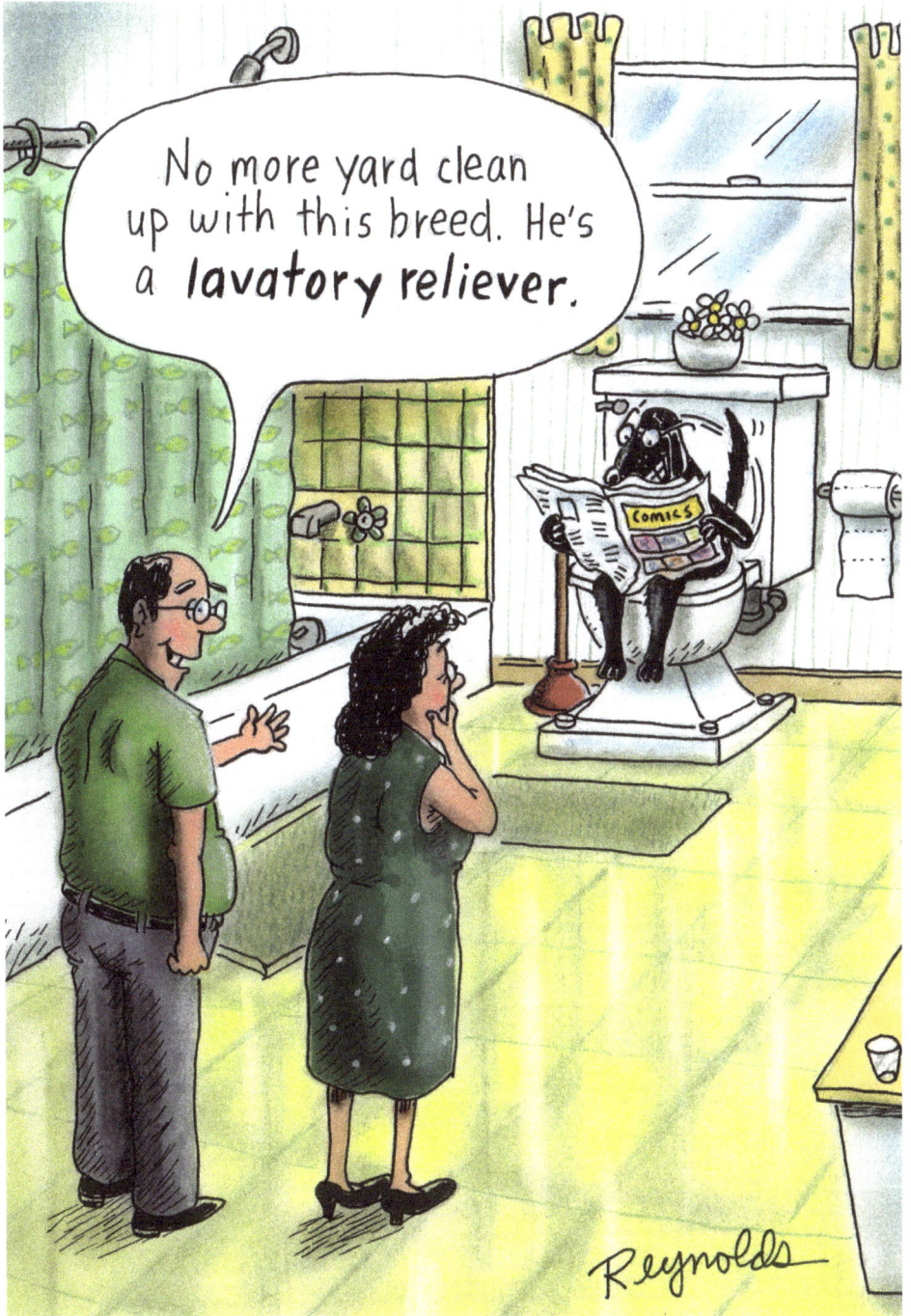

The Bark Side: It's a Dog's Life!

Dogs are omnivores, which means they feed on a wide variety of foods including meat, vegetables and grains.

Apart from barking, growling and whining, dogs use their ears and facial expression to communicate what they are feeling.

Puppies are born blind, without teeth and the ability to hear. Their eyes only open at around 10 to 14 days old, and their hearing will start after this. Their teeth start coming through at 6 weeks.

During the first week of a dog's life, 90% of their time is spent sleeping, and 10% is spent eating.

Puppies are considered adults when they are one year old.

The fastest dog on earth can reach speeds of 45 miles an hour, and is the Greyhound.

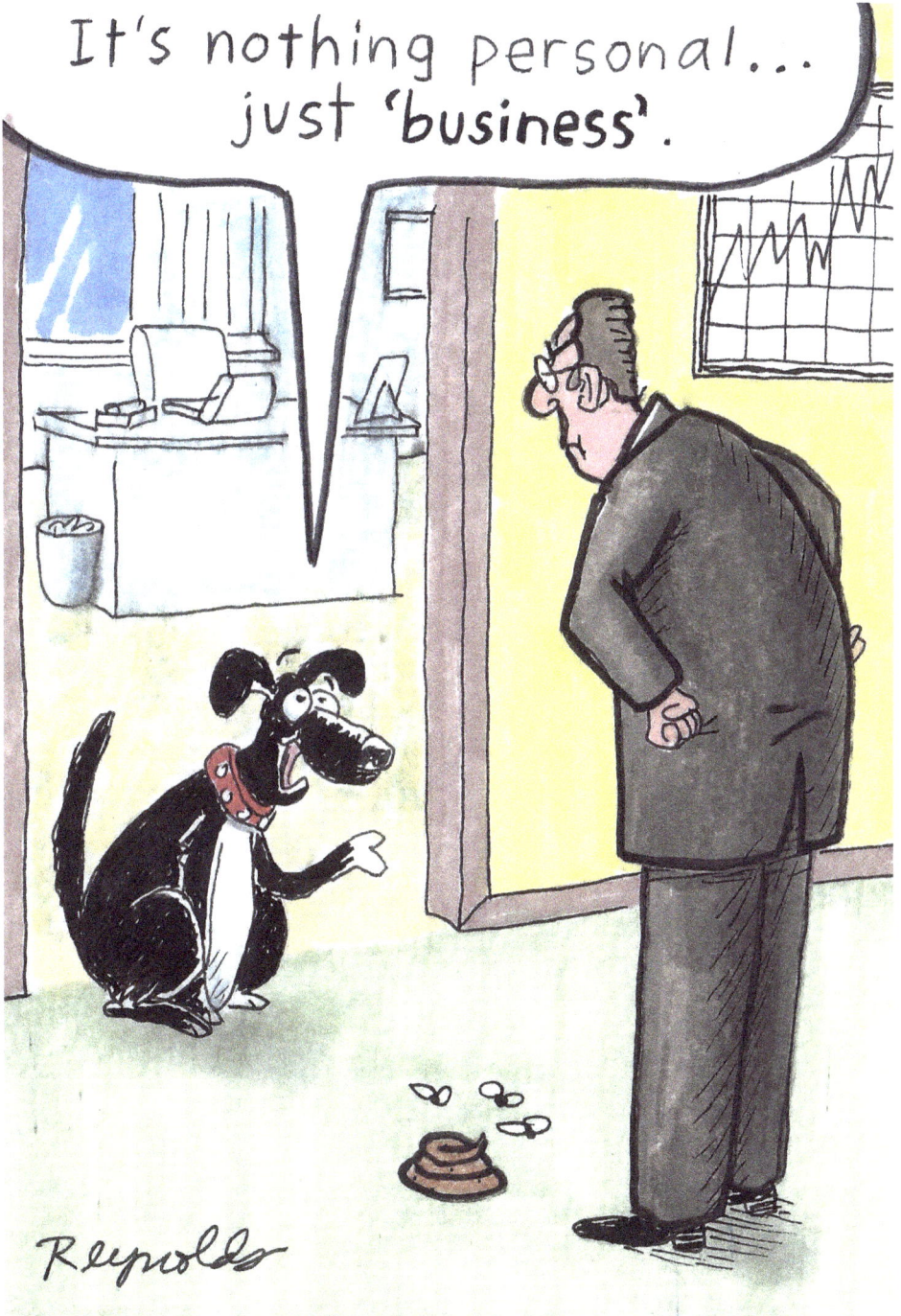

The Bark Side: It's a Dog's Life!

The domestic dog is a descendant of the grey wolf, in a process that took around 100,000 years.

The nickname "man's best friend" is believed to have come from a courtroom speech in Missouri America in 1870 where a farmer was suing his neighbor who shot his dog.

The very first animal to go into space was a dog, a Russian dog named Laika who travelled in the spacecraft Sputnik around the earth in 1957.

Some dogs change colors as they grow, like Dalmatians which are born white and then develop black spots as they mature. Airedales are similar, born completely black they will grow grey, black and tan fur as they get older.

The Beagle and the Border Collie are the dogs that bark the most.

The Bark Side: It's a Dog's Life!

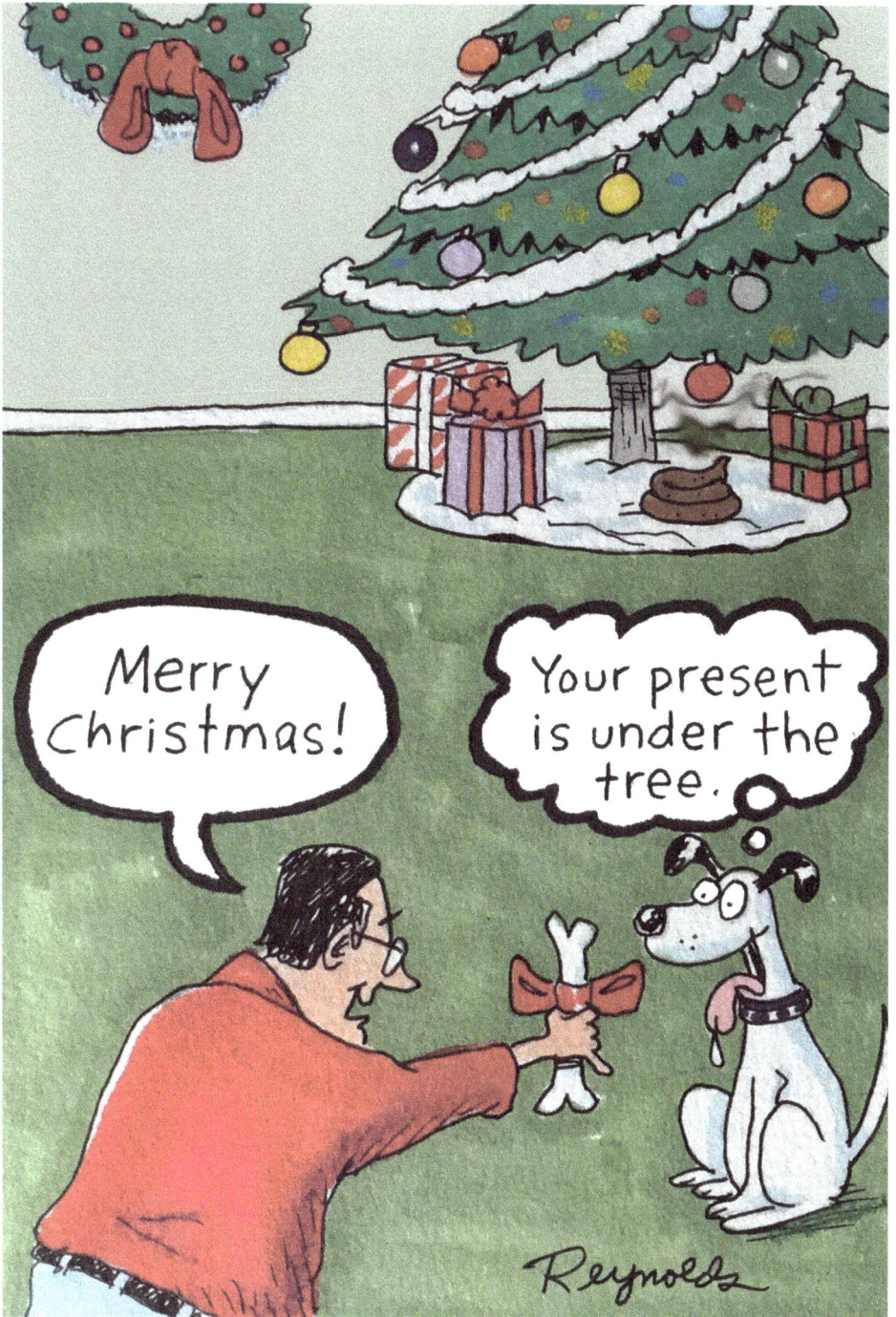

The Bark Side: It's a Dog's Life!

Dogs should not eat raisins, grapes, onion, chocolate or garlic because it makes them very sick.

To many dogs showing a smile (baring your teeth) is an act of aggression. Most dogs don't smile with their mouths like people do, but show happiness and excitement by wagging their tails.

Dogs see much better than humans at night because they have a special light reflecting layer behind their eyes.

There is a hunting dog that comes from Africa that cannot bark, it is the only dog like this and the sound is makes is commonly known as 'barroo'.

The world record for the heaviest dog ever recorded was set in 1989, an Old English Mastiff that weighed 343 pounds and was 8 feet 3 inches long.

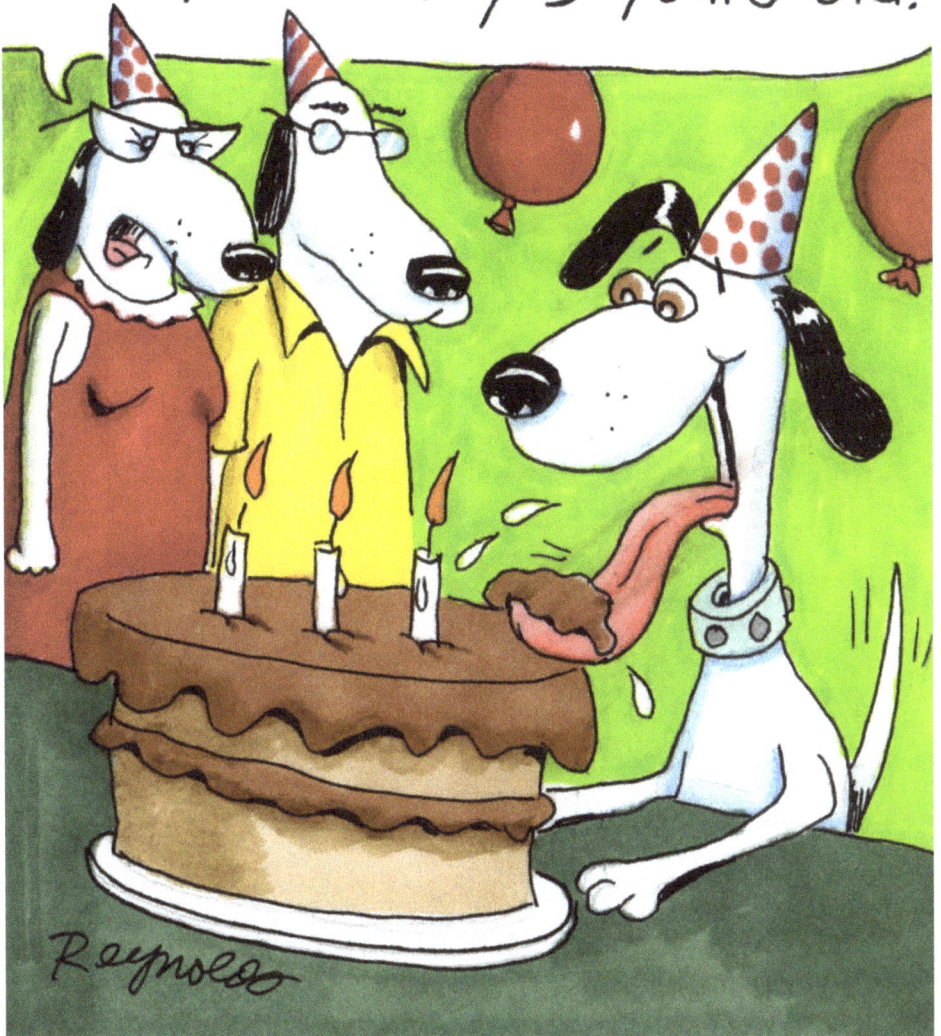

Dogs hearts beat much faster than ours, between 10-120 beats a minute while humans are 70-80.

Small dogs are often called toy dogs, or lap dogs – because they're so small they look like a toy, or can easily fit on your lap.

The first thing you should teach your dog is how to 'sit'.

A dog's vision is not as good as a human's, and they are much better at seeing moving objects rather than those standing still. If you're 300 yards away from your dog they will be unable to see you, until you wave your arms or move around.

The largest breed of dog in the world is the Irish Wolfhound, and the smallest dog breed is the Chihuahua. St. Bernard's are the heaviest breed of dogs.

The Bark Side: It's a Dog's Life!

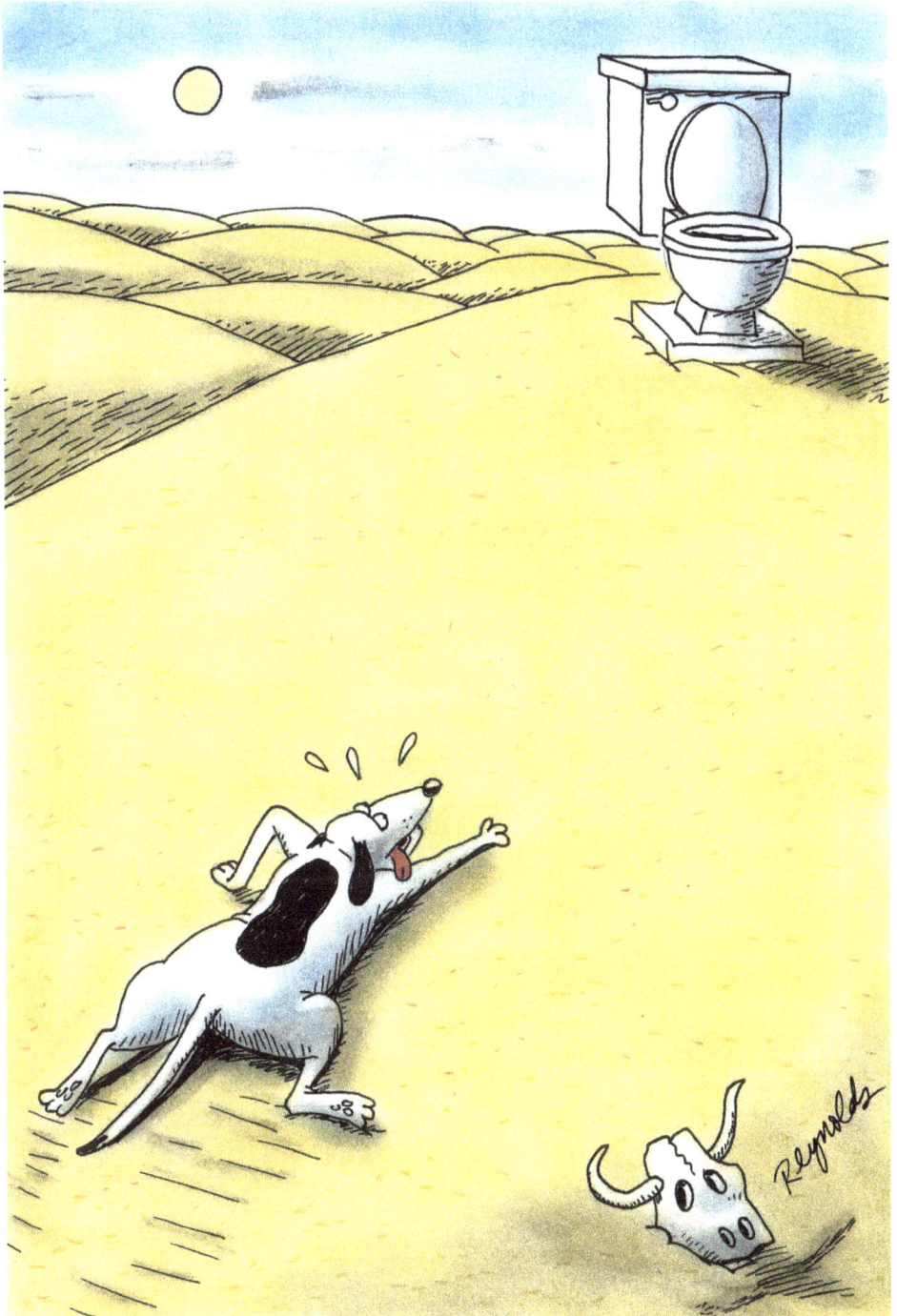

The Bark Side: It's a Dog's Life!

The oldest dog who ever lived was a cattle dog from Australia called Bluey who lived to be 29 years and 5 months old. In human terms that makes him over 160 years old!

When your dog goes to sleep you notice he turns in a circle a few times, this is an instinct from when they were a wild dog, as they did this to pat down the grass before they slept. Despite thousands of years, they still have this instinct.

If your puppy takes something you don't want them to have, don't chase them. Instead make it a game where they chase you (and you run away) and you'll have the item back in no time.

The rock star Ozzy Osborne rescued his wife's Pomeranian from a coyote by wrestling the coyote until it released the dog.

The Bark Side: It's a Dog's Life!

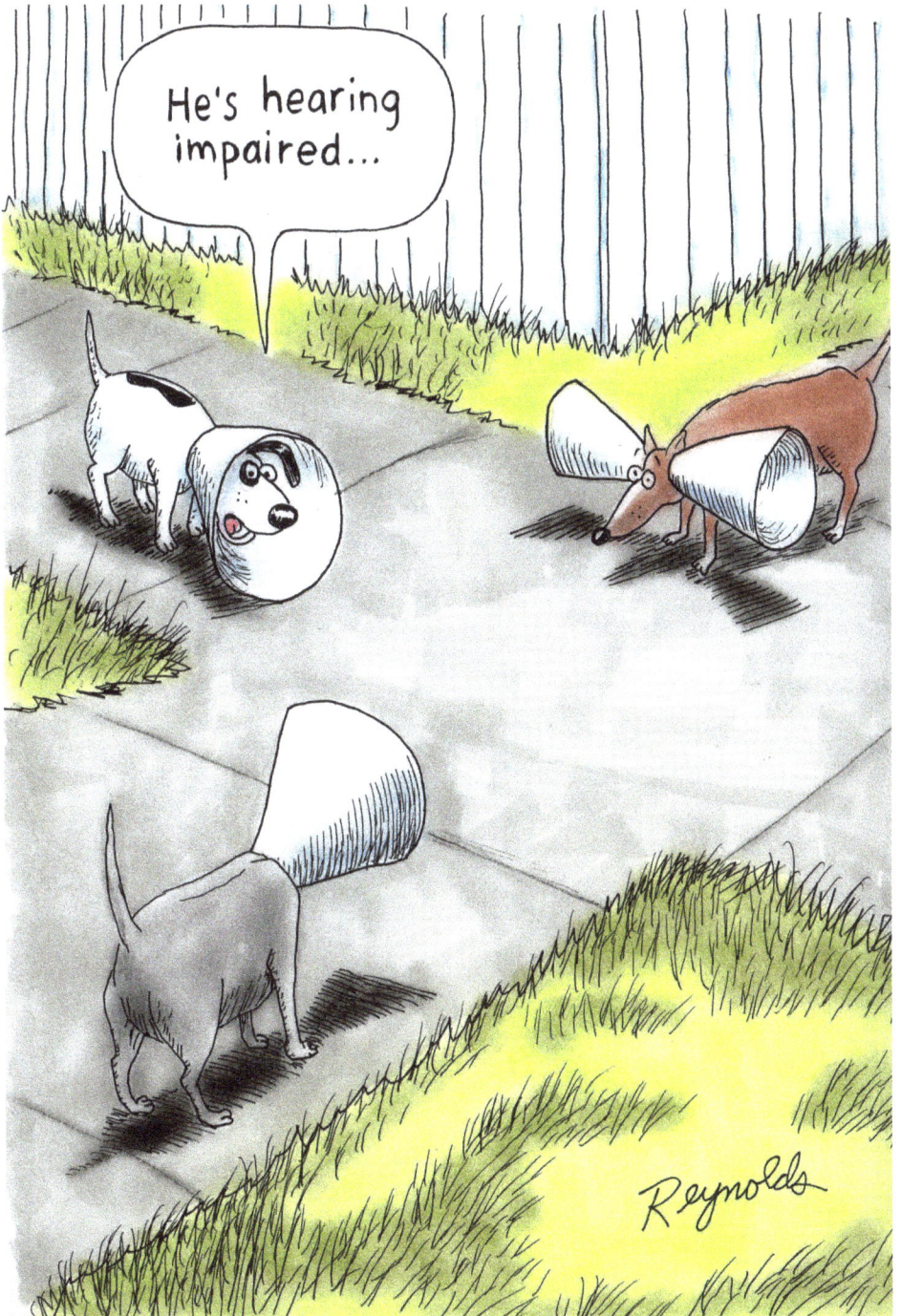

The Bark Side: It's a Dog's Life!

The most dogs ever owned by a single person was 5,000 Mastiffs which were owned by Kubla Khan.

The weirdest law about dogs is that in Paulding, Ohio police officers are allowed to bite a dog to get it to be quiet.

In Iran, it is against the law to own a dog as a pet, you need to be able to prove they are a guard or hunting dog.

There are cave paintings of dogs in Spain in Europe that are over 12,000 years old.

Even the presidents love their dogs, and President Franklin Roosevelt sent a destroyer to the Aleutian Islands just to get his dog Fala, who had been left behind.

A dog's nose print is unique, and similar to human fingerprints that no two are the same.

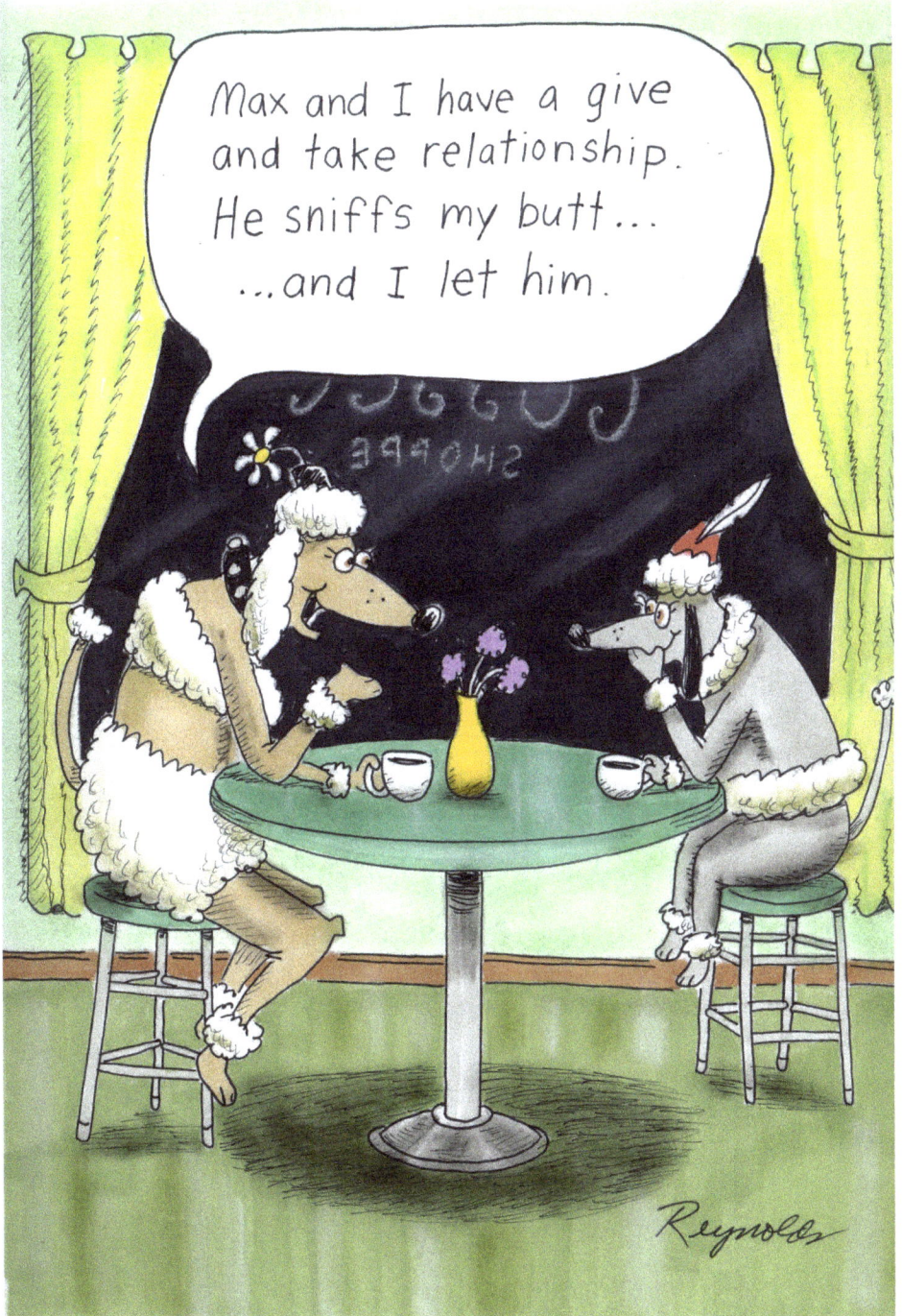

The Bark Side: It's a Dog's Life!

According to ancient Greek literature, when Odysseus arrived home after an absence of 20 years, disguised as a beggar, the only one to recognize him was his aged dog Argos, who wagged his tail at his master, and then died.

The expression "three dog night" originated with the Eskimos and means a very cold night - so cold that you have to bed down with three dogs to keep warm.

An American Animal Hospital Association poll showed that 33 percent of dog owners admit that they talk to their dogs on the phone or leave messages on an answering machine while away.

Seventy percent of people sign their pet's name on greeting cards and 58 percent include their pets in family and holiday portraits, according to a survey done by the American Animal Hospital Association.

The Bark Side: It's a Dog's Life!

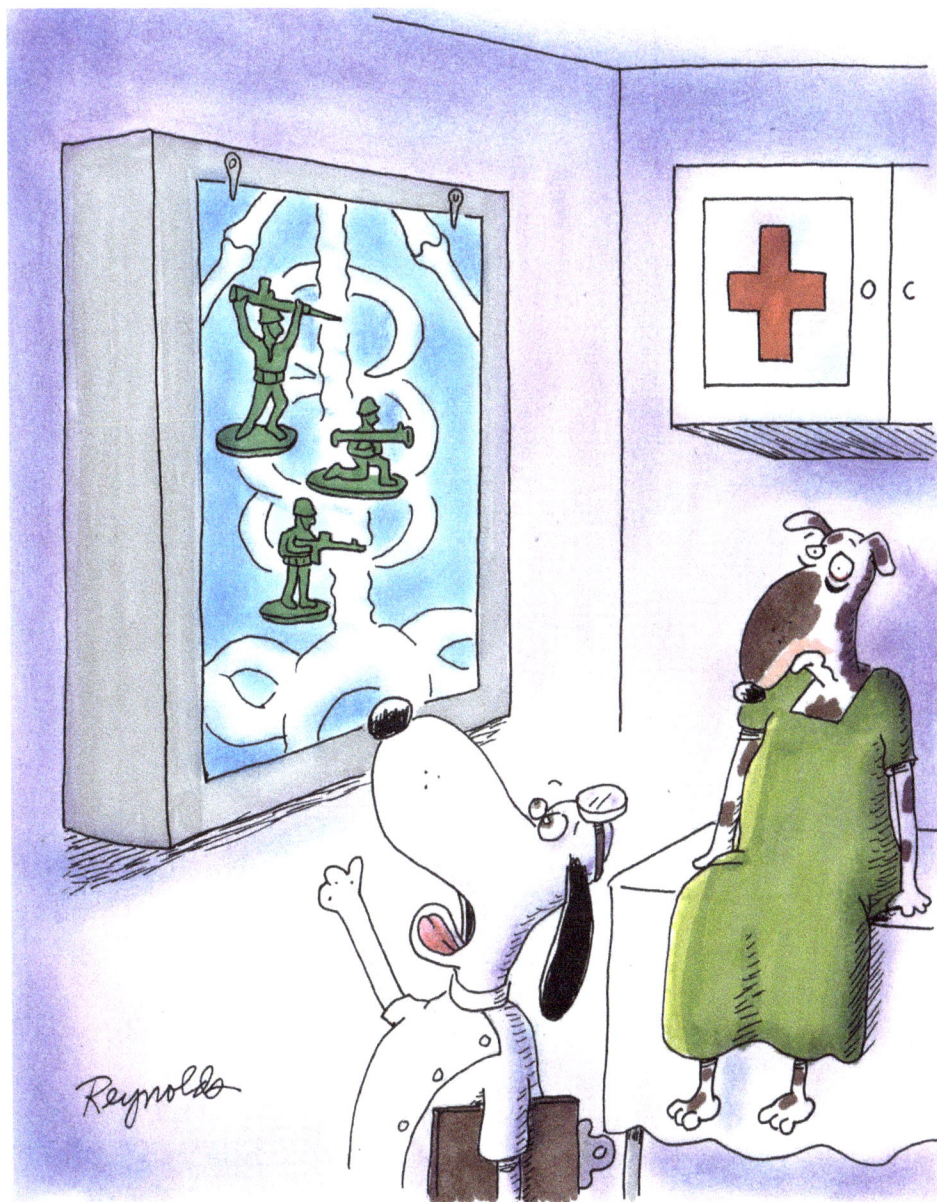

"The bad news is you've swallowed a bunch of those little, green plastic army soldiers. The good news is they all ended up in your *G.I.* tract."

The Bark Side: It's a Dog's Life!

There are 701 types of pure breed dogs. The smallest breed of dog recognized by the American Kennel Club is the Chihuahua, which stands six to nine inches at the top of the shoulders and weighs two to six pounds. The largest is the Irish Wolfhound, which stands 30 to 35 inches at the top of the shoulders and weighs 105 to 125 pounds.

Pekingese dogs were sacred to the emperors of China for more than 2,000 years. They are one of the oldest breeds of dogs in the world.

Bloodhound dogs have the best sense of smell of all dogs, and have been used to track down criminals since the middle ages.

A survey found that 33% of dog owners talk to their dogs on the phone when they are away, or leave messages on the answering machine.

The Bark Side: It's a Dog's Life!

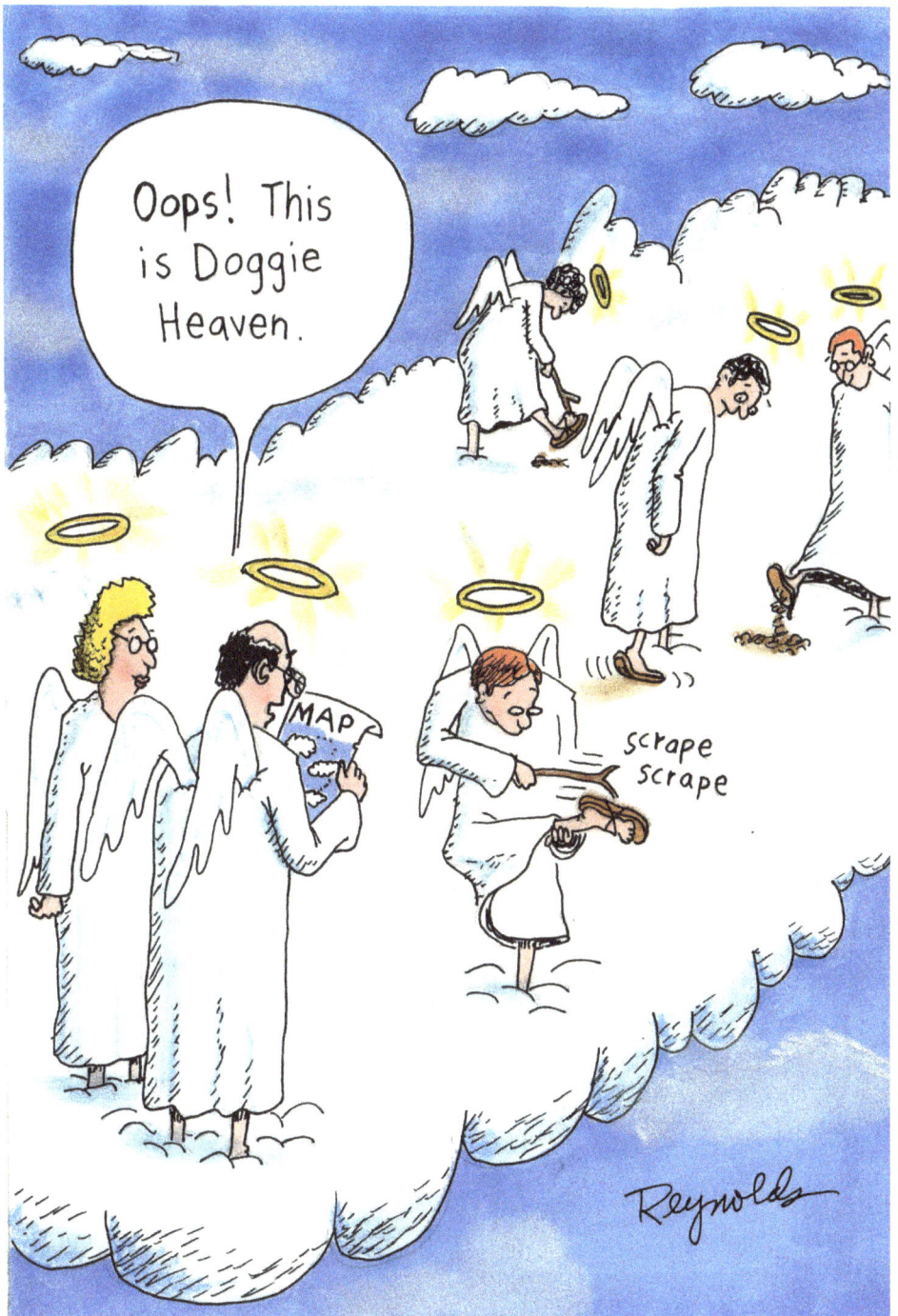

While small dogs are gaining in popularity, the top dogs are still the big ones. The Labrador Retriever, Golden Retriever, and German Shepherd Dog are first, second, and third on list of the American Kennel Club's most popular breeds.

Scientists have discovered that dogs can smell the presence of autism in children. "Seizure Alert" dogs can alert their owners up to an hour before the onset of an epileptic seizure.

Bad breath can be a sign of tarter buildup and bacteria. To reduce odor, brush your dog's teeth, and take him to the vet for routine dental cleanings.

Many people believe dogs that crouch or lower their heads when approached have been abused, but some dogs are so submissive that they naturally behave this way.

The Bark Side: It's a Dog's Life!

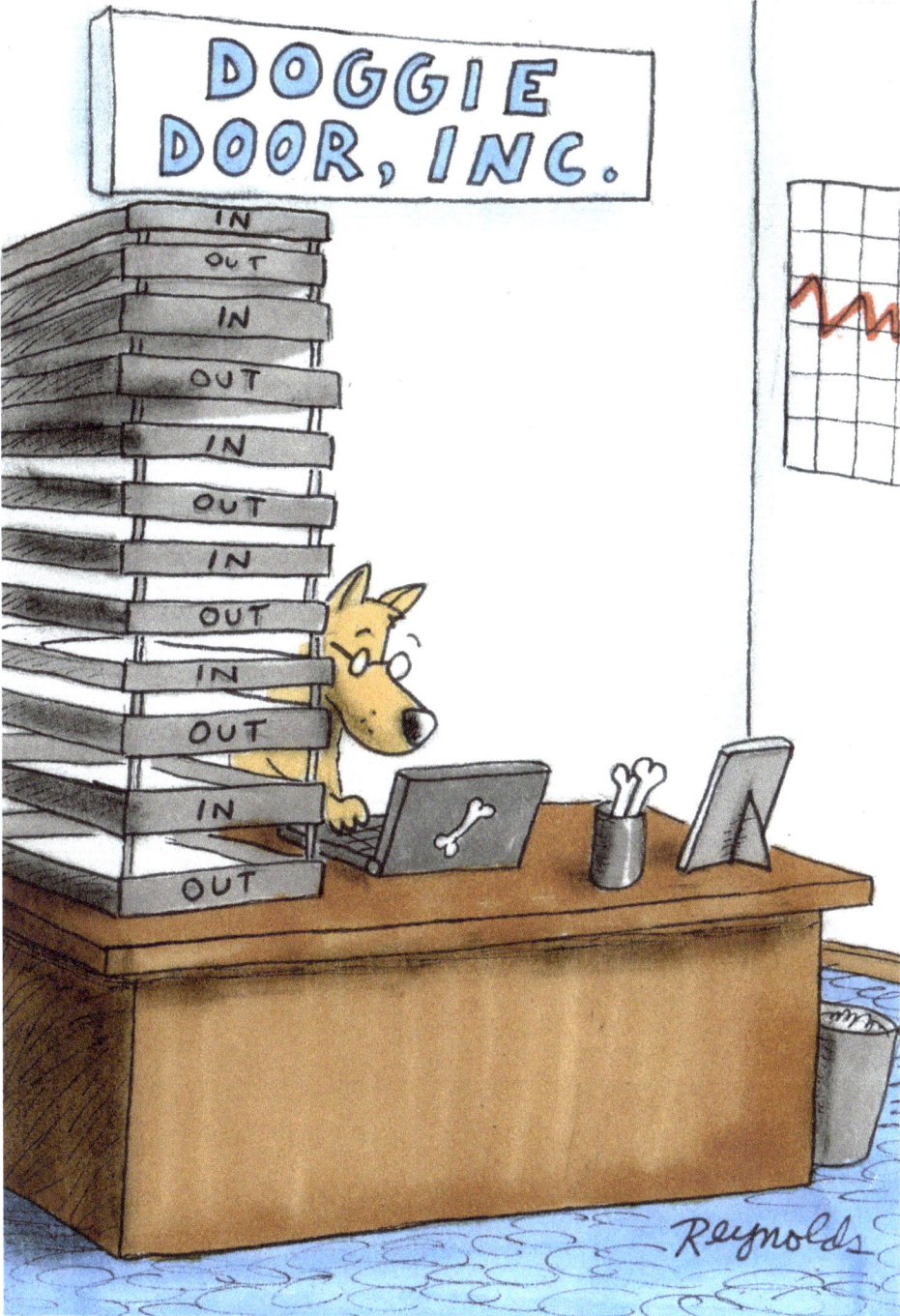

The Bark Side: It's a Dog's Life!

If your dog requires professional dog grooming try and choose a company that specializes in your dog breed. You will find that your dog will look so much better if you find someone who knows their job.

Dogs reserve their tail wags for living things. A dog will wag its tail for a person, or another dog and may do so for a cat, horse, mouse or even a moth. If the dog is alone, however, it does not wag its tail.

The theobromine in chocolate that stimulates the cardiac and nervous systems is too much for dogs, especially smaller pups. A chocolate bar is poisonous to dogs and can even be lethal.

Though human noses have an impressive 5 million olfactory cells with which to smell, sheepdogs have 220 million, enabling them to smell 44 times better than man.

The Bark Side: It's a Dog's Life!

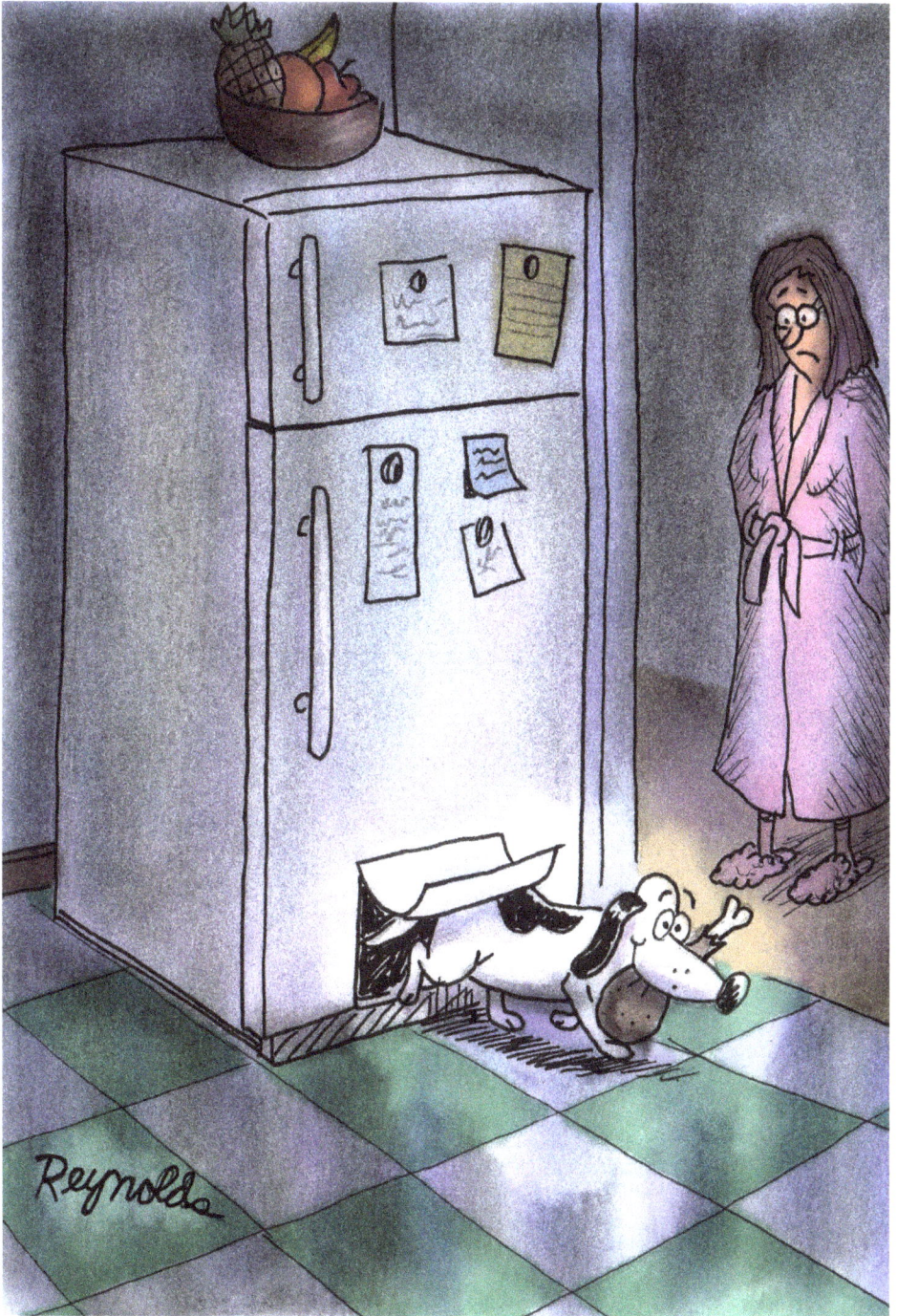

The common belief that dogs are color blind is false. Dogs can see color, but it is not as vivid a color scheme as we see. They distinguish between blue, yellow, and gray, but probably do not see red and green. This is much like our vision at twilight.

Using their swiveling ears like radar dishes, experiments have shown that dogs can locate the source of a sound in 6/100ths of a second.

A dog's heart beats between 70 and 120 times a minute, compared with a human heart which beats 70 to 80 times a minute.

A dog's normal body temperature is 100.5 to 102.5 degrees Fahrenheit.

A female carries her young about 60 days before the puppies are born.

The Bark Side: It's a Dog's Life!

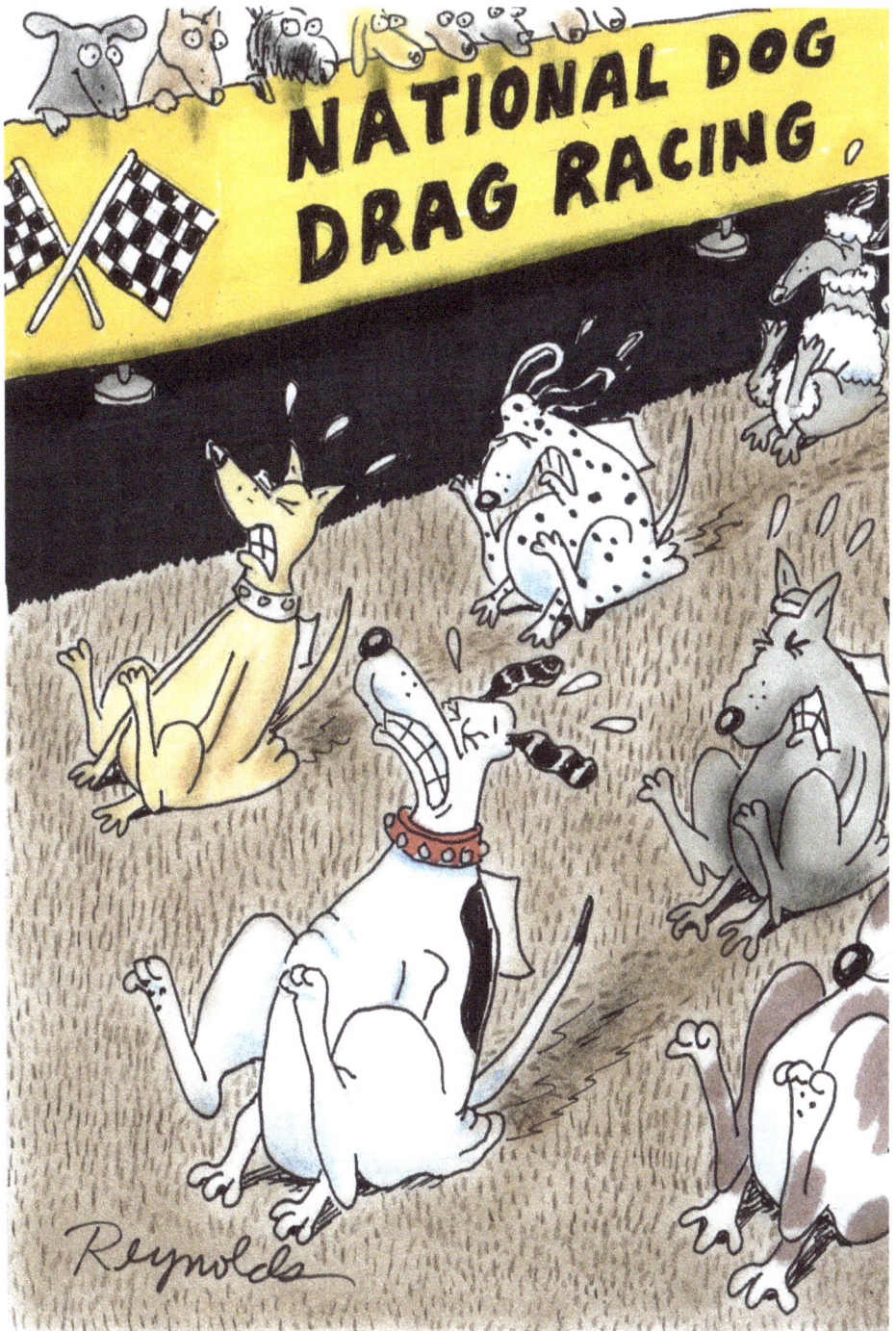

According to the Guinness Book of World Records, the smallest dog on record was a Yorkshire Terrier in Great Britain who, at the age of 2, weighed just 4 ounces.

The longest-lived dog, according to the Guinness Book of World Records, was an Australian Cattle Dog, named Bluey, who lived to be 29.

An adult dog has 42 teeth.

The best time to train your dog is from the day you bring it home regardless of its age. Use positive rewards and ignore bad behavior. When your dog does something good then reward it. If it does something bad, like jumping up on you, then ignore it.

It is a myth that dogs are color blind. They can actually see in color, just not as vividly as humans. It is akin to our vision at dusk.

The Bark Side: It's a Dog's Life!

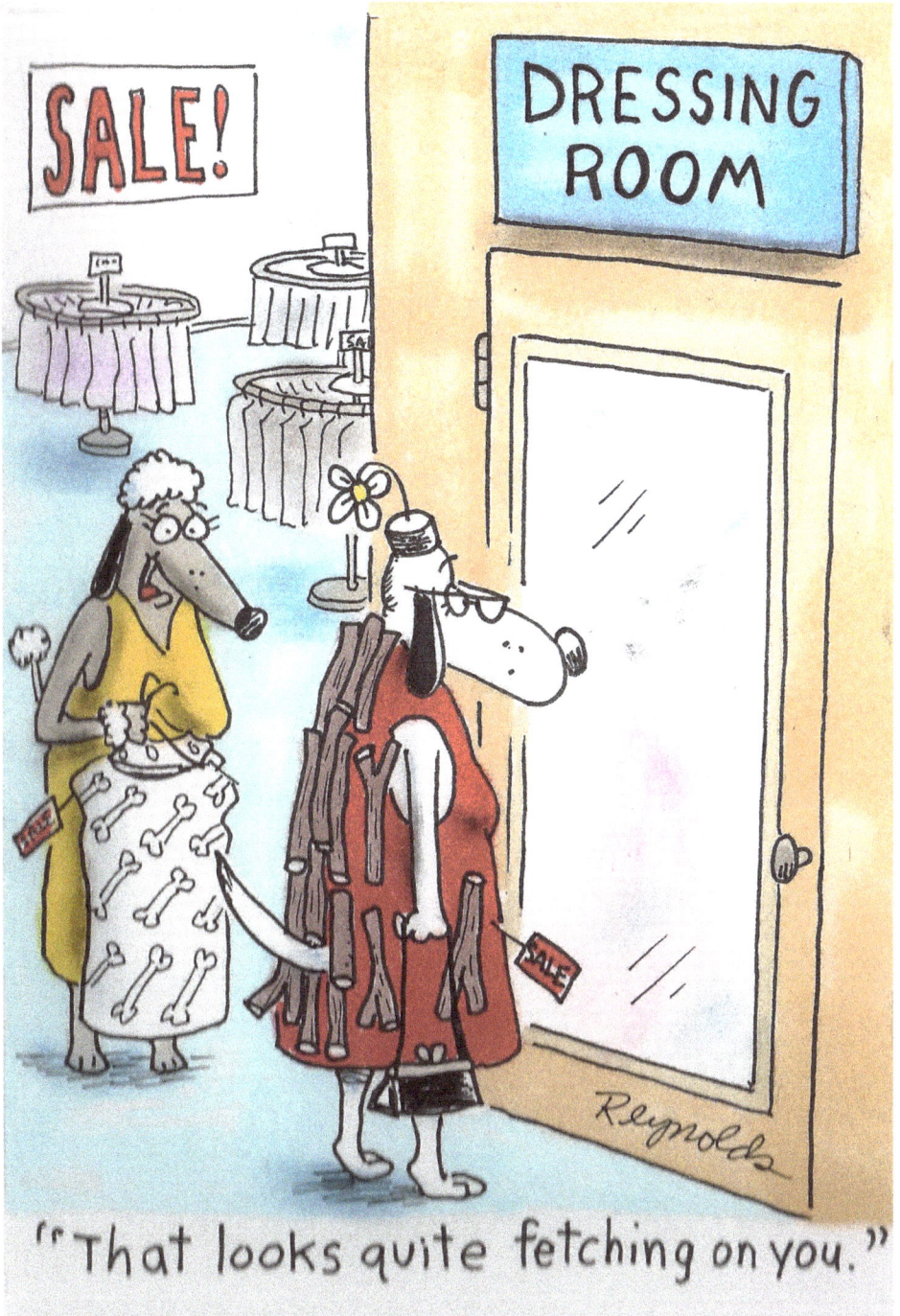

"That looks quite fetching on you."

The Bark Side: It's a Dog's Life!

If never spayed or neutered, a female dog, her mate, and their puppies could produce over 66,000 dogs in 6 years!

The only sweat glands a dog has are between the paw pads.

In 1957, Laika became the first living being in space via an earth satellite.

The world's smartest dogs are thought to be (1) the border collie, (2) the poodle, and (3) the golden retriever.

Chocolate contains a substance known as theobromine (similar to caffeine) which can kill dogs or at the very least make them violently ill.

Dogs' sense of hearing is more than ten times more acute than a human's

More than 1 in 3 American families own a dog.

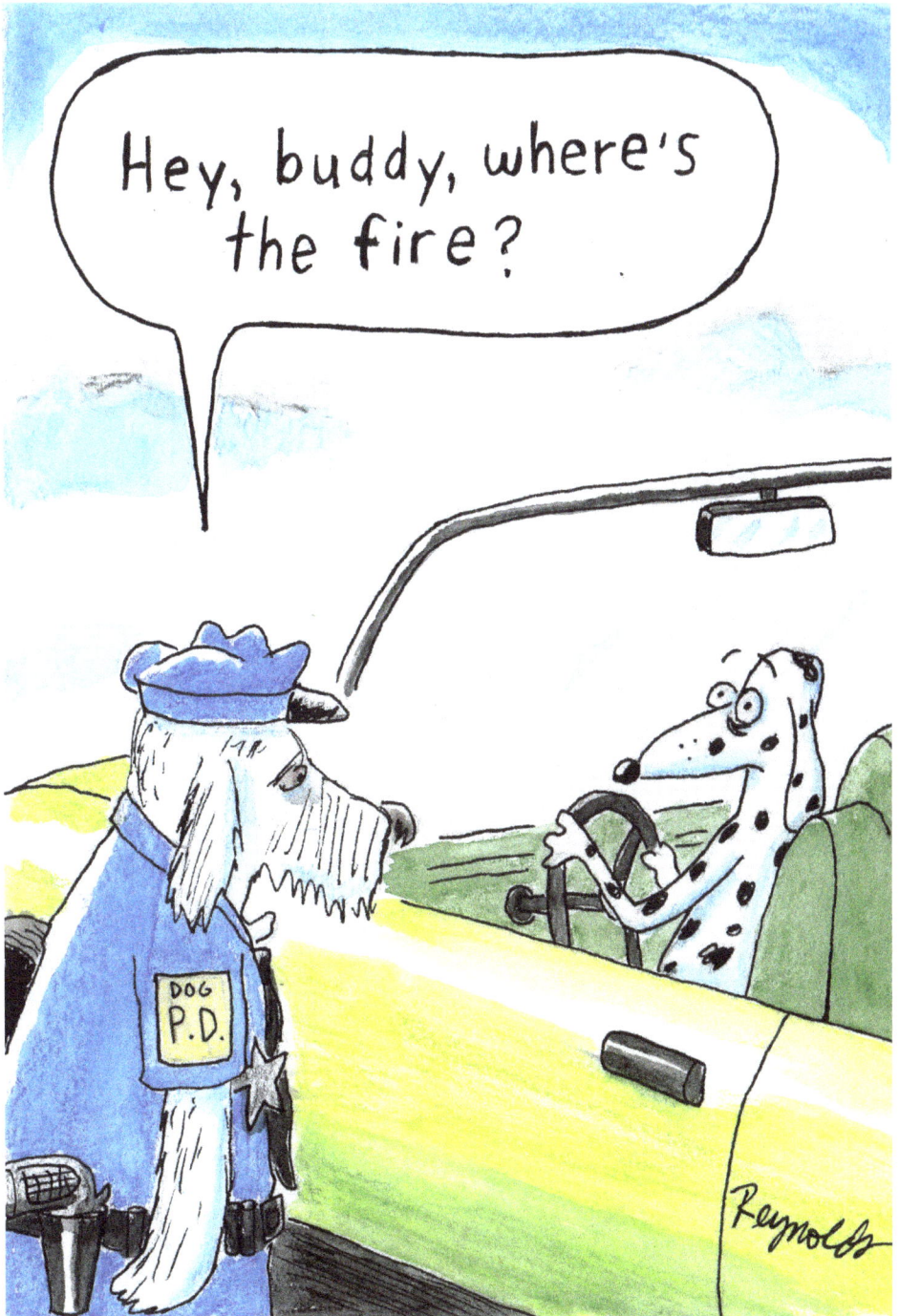

The Bark Side: It's a Dog's Life!

Dogs don't like rain because the sound is amplified and hurts their very sensitive ears.

The ten most popular dogs (AKC, 2007) are in order: Labrador Retriever, Yorkshire Terrier, German Shepherd, Golden Retriever, Beagle, Boxer, Dachshund, Poodle, Shih Tzu, and Bulldog.

Dogs were the first animals domesticated by people.

A greyhound can run as fast as 45 miles an hour.

Spaying/neutering your dog before the age of 6 months can help prevent cancer in your dog.

Puppies acquire a full mouth of permanent teeth between four and seven months old.

The Bark Side: It's a Dog's Life!

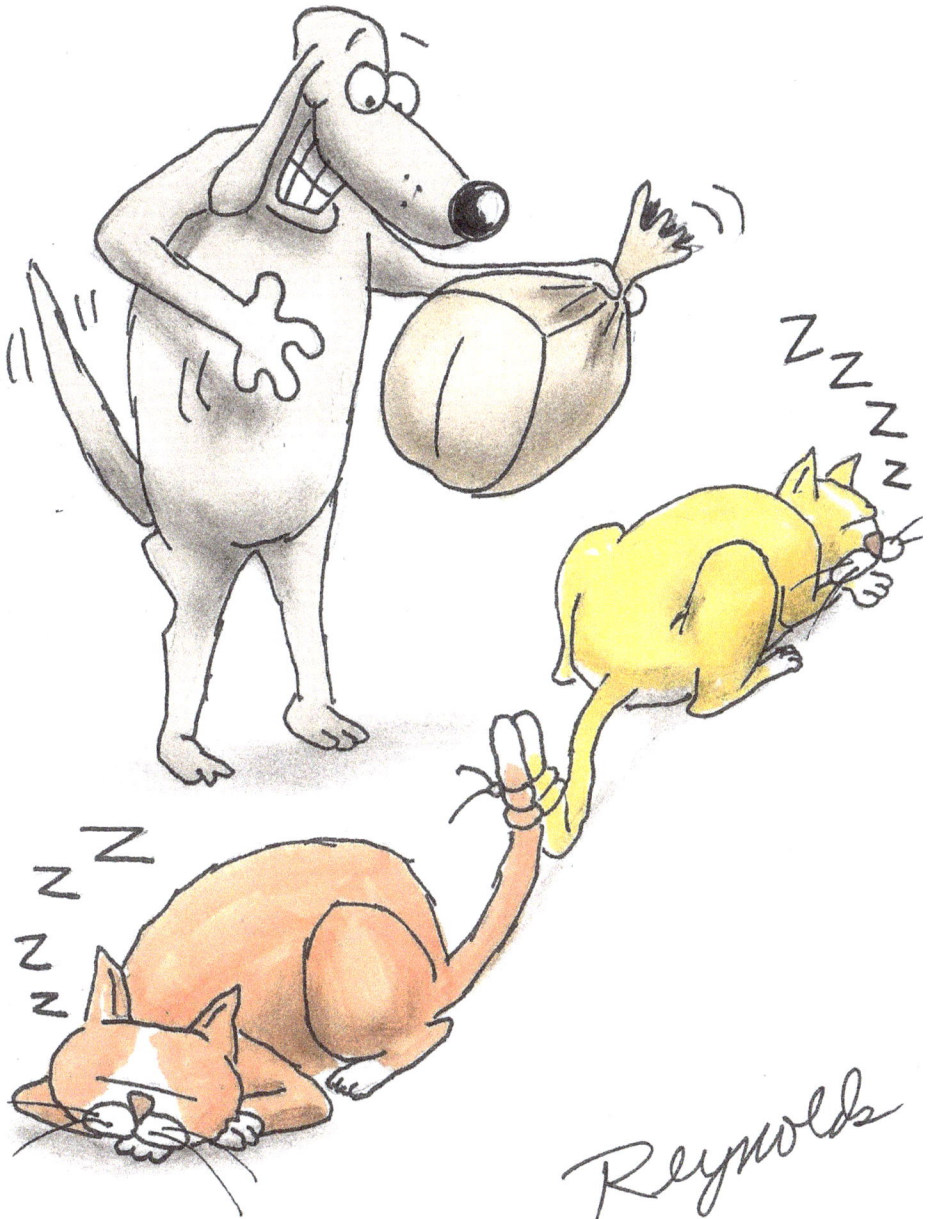

The Bark Side: It's a Dog's Life!

Small dogs live the longest. Toy breeds live up to 16 years or more. Larger dogs average is 7 – 12 years. Veterinary medicine has extended this estimate by about three years. However, some breeds, such as Tibetan terrier live as long as twenty years.

Eighty percent of dog owners buy their dog a present for holidays and birthdays. More than half of them sign letters and cards from themselves and their pets.

Most pet owners (94 percent) say their pet makes them smile more than once a day.

All dogs can be traced back 40 million years ago to a weasel-like animal called the Miacis which dwelled in trees and dens. The Miacis later evolved into the Tomarctus, a direct forbearer of the genus Canis, which includes the wolf and jackal as well as the dog.

The Bark Side: It's a Dog's Life!

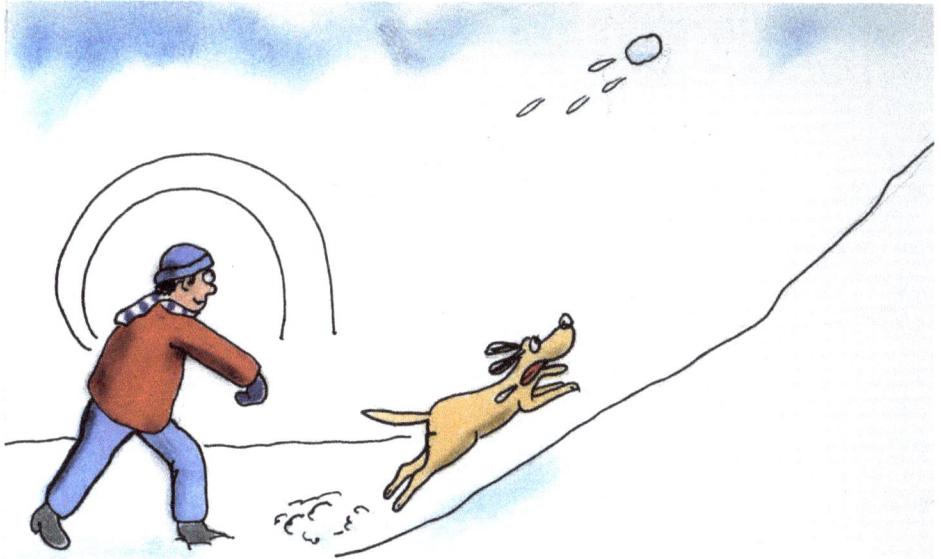

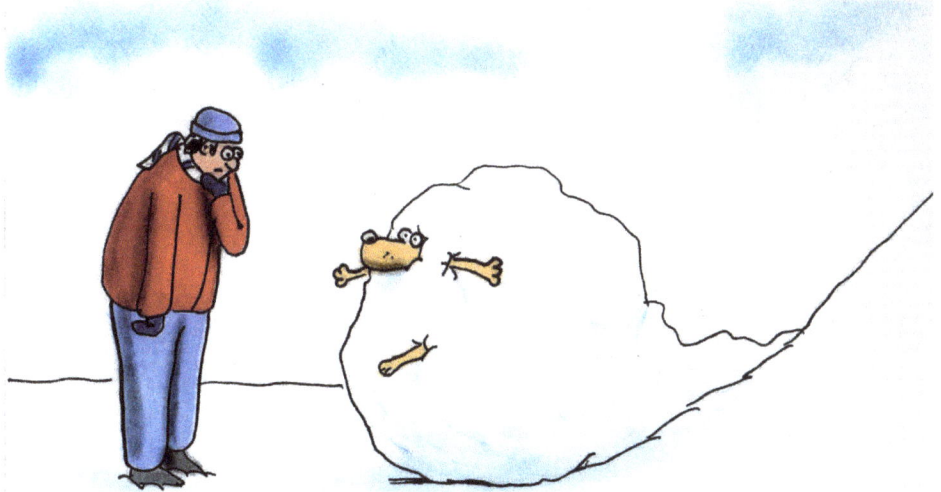

The Bark Side: It's a Dog's Life!

The dog name "Fido" is from Latin and means "fidelity."

The U.S. has the highest dog population in the world.

It has been established that people who own pets live longer, have less stress, and have fewer heart attacks.

Dogs are mentioned 14 times in the Bible.

Seventy percent of people sign their pet's name on greeting cards and 58 percent include their pets in family and holiday portraits, according to a survey done by the American Animal Hospital Association.

A dog's whiskers are touch-sensitive hairs called vibrissae. They are found on the muzzle, above the eyes and below the jaws, and can actually sense tiny changes in airflow.

The Bark Side: It's a Dog's Life!

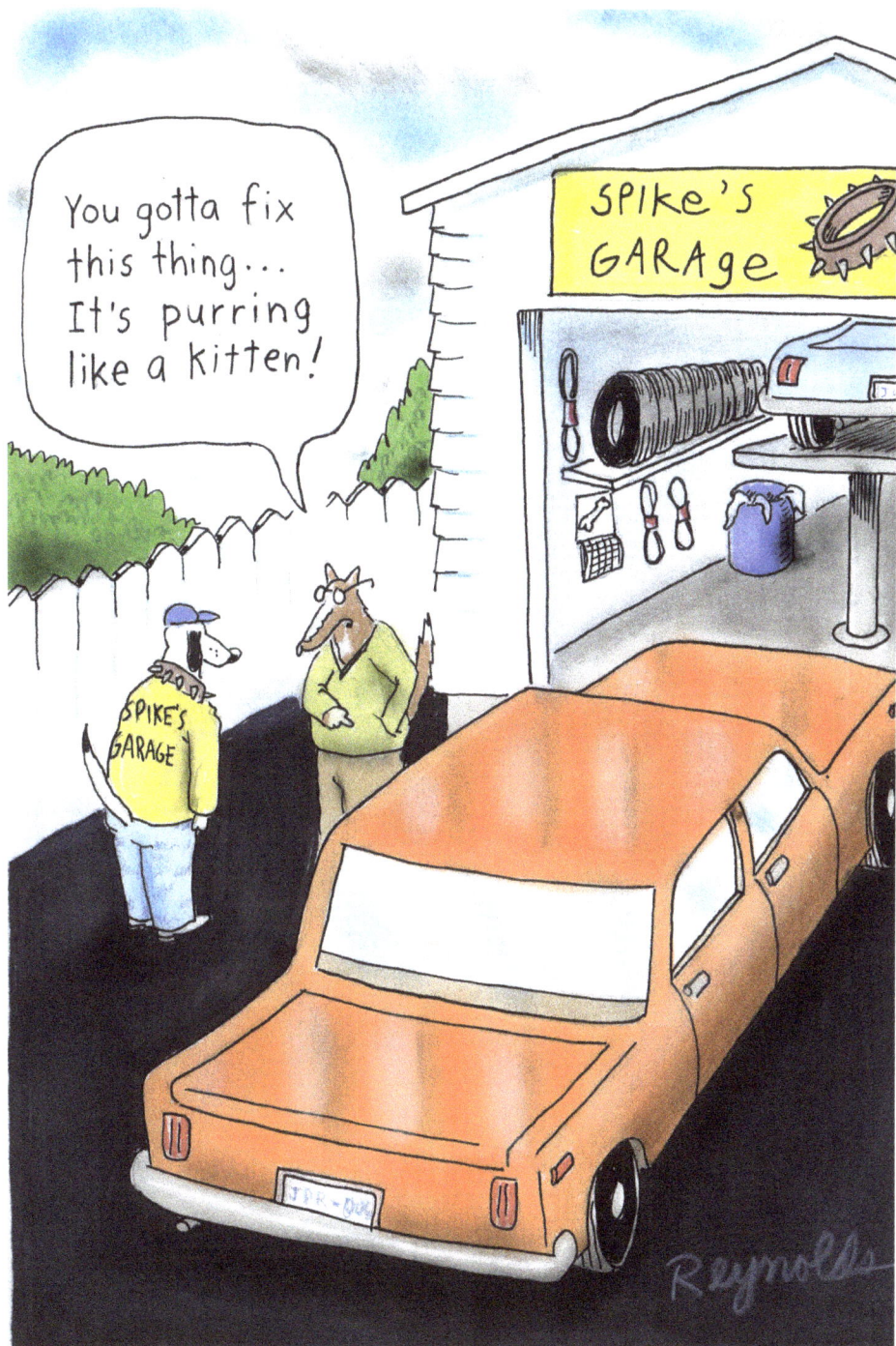

The origin of amputating a dog's tail may go back to the Roman writer Lucius Columella's (A.D. 4-70) assertion that tail docking prevented rabies.

Dogs can smell about 1,000 times better than humans. While humans have 5 million smell-detecting cells, dogs have more than 220 million. The part of the brain that interprets smell is also four times larger in dogs than in humans.

The Labrador Retriever has been on the AKC's top 10 most popular breeds list for 25 consecutive years—longer than any other breed.

A dog's nose print is unique, much like a person's fingerprint.

Forty-five percent of U.S. dogs sleep in their owner's bed.

The Bark Side: It's a Dog's Life!

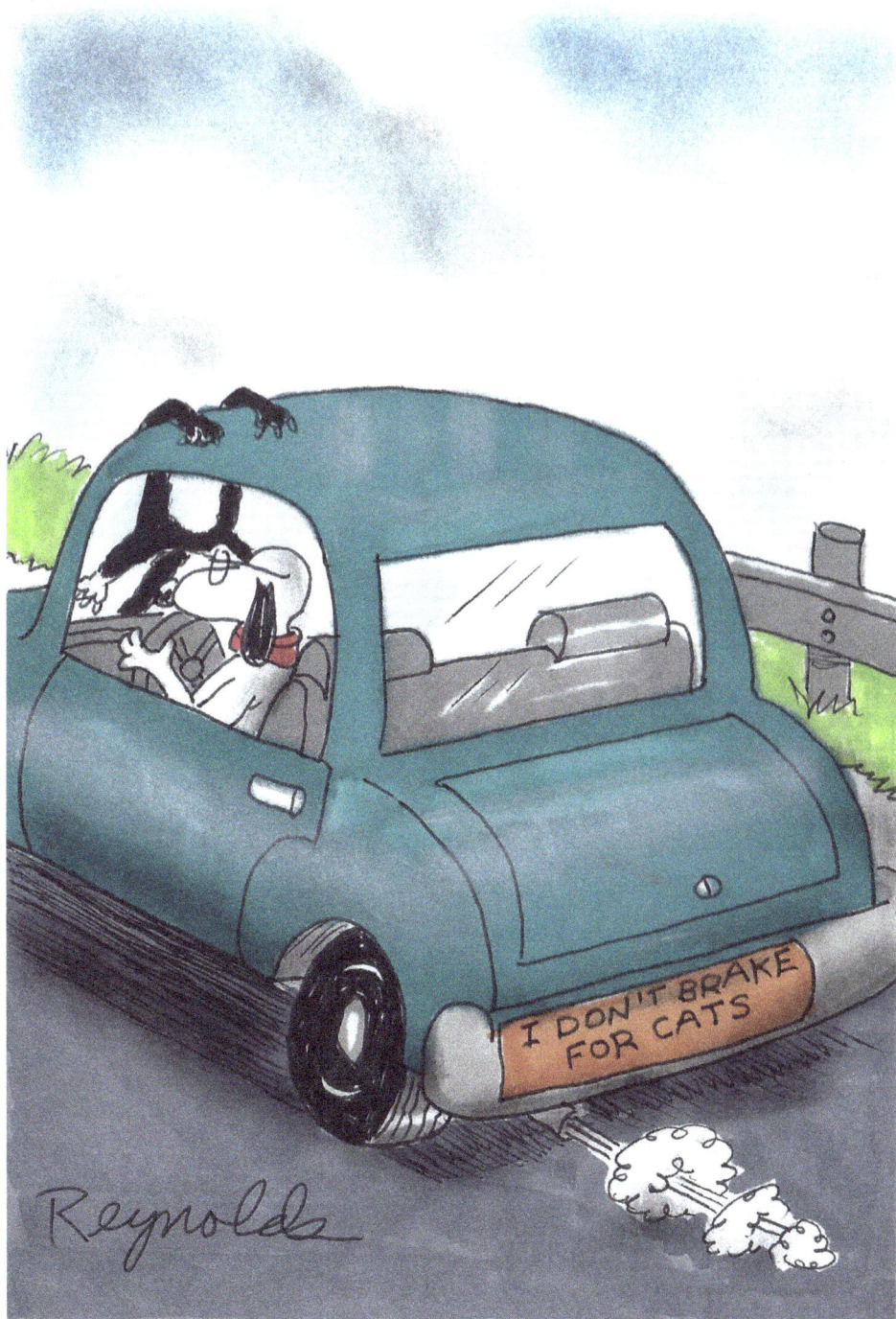

Speaking of sleeping ... all dogs dream, but puppies and senior dogs dream more frequently than adult dogs.

Seventy percent of people sign their dog's name on their holiday cards.

A dog's sense of smell is legendary, but did you know that his nose has as many as 300 million receptors? In comparison, a human nose has about 5 million.

Rin Tin Tin, the famous German Shepherd, was nominated for an Academy Award.

The shape of a dog's face suggests its longevity: A long face means a longer life.

Dog eyes have a part called the *tapetum lucidum*, allowing night vision.

The name Collie means "black." (Collies once tended black-faced sheep.)

The Bark Side: It's a Dog's Life!

Herding dog
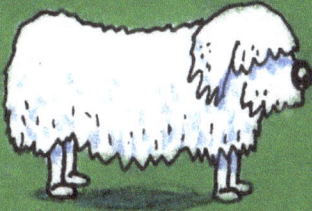

Guard dog
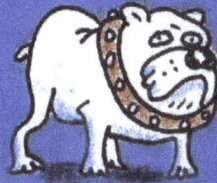

Hunting dog
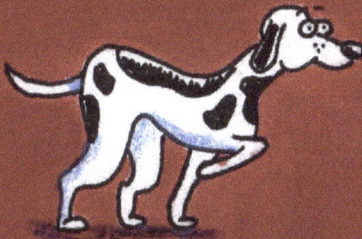

Lap dog
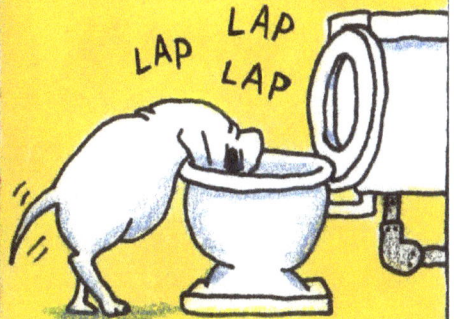

Dog Breeds

Yawning is contagious—even for dogs. Research shows that the sound of a human yawn can trigger one from your dog. And it's four times as likely to happen when it's the yawn of a person he knows.

The Dandie Dinmont Terrier is the only breed named for a fictional person—a character in the novel *Guy Mannering*, by Sir Walter Scott.

Dogs curl up in a ball when sleeping to protect their organs—a hold over from their days in the wild, when they were vulnerable to predator attacks.

The Basenji is not technically "barkless," as many people think. They can yodel.

The Australian Shepherd is not actually from Australia—they are an American breed.

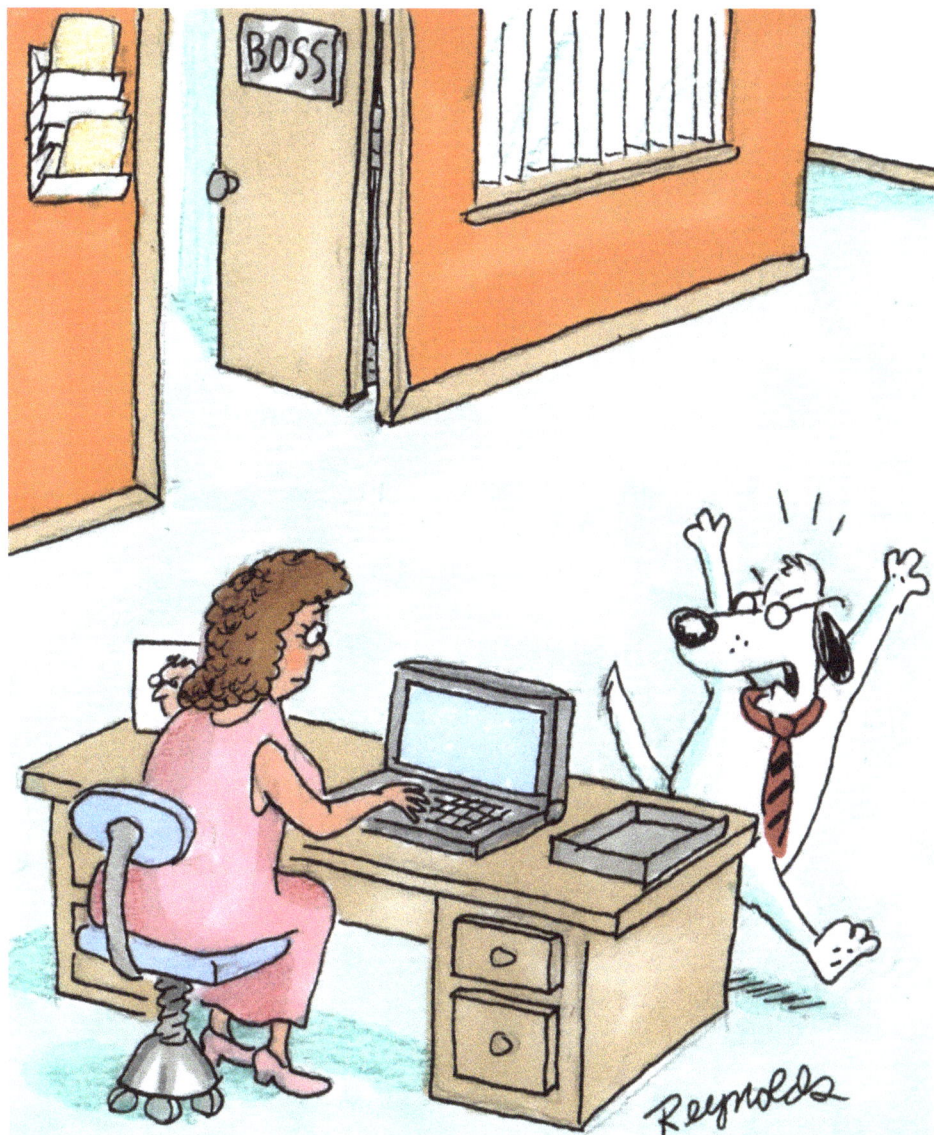

"A raise? Huh! He won't even throw me a bone!"

The Bark Side: It's a Dog's Life!

The Labrador Retriever is originally from Newfoundland.

Human blood pressure goes down when petting a dog. And so does the dog's.

There are over 75 million pet dogs in the U.S.—more than in any other country.

A person who hunts with a Beagle is known as a "Beagler."

Dogs are not colorblind. They also see blue and yellow.

All puppies are born deaf.

Dalmatians are born completely white, and develop their spots as they get older.

Dogs have about 1,700 taste buds. (We humans have between 2,000–10,000.)

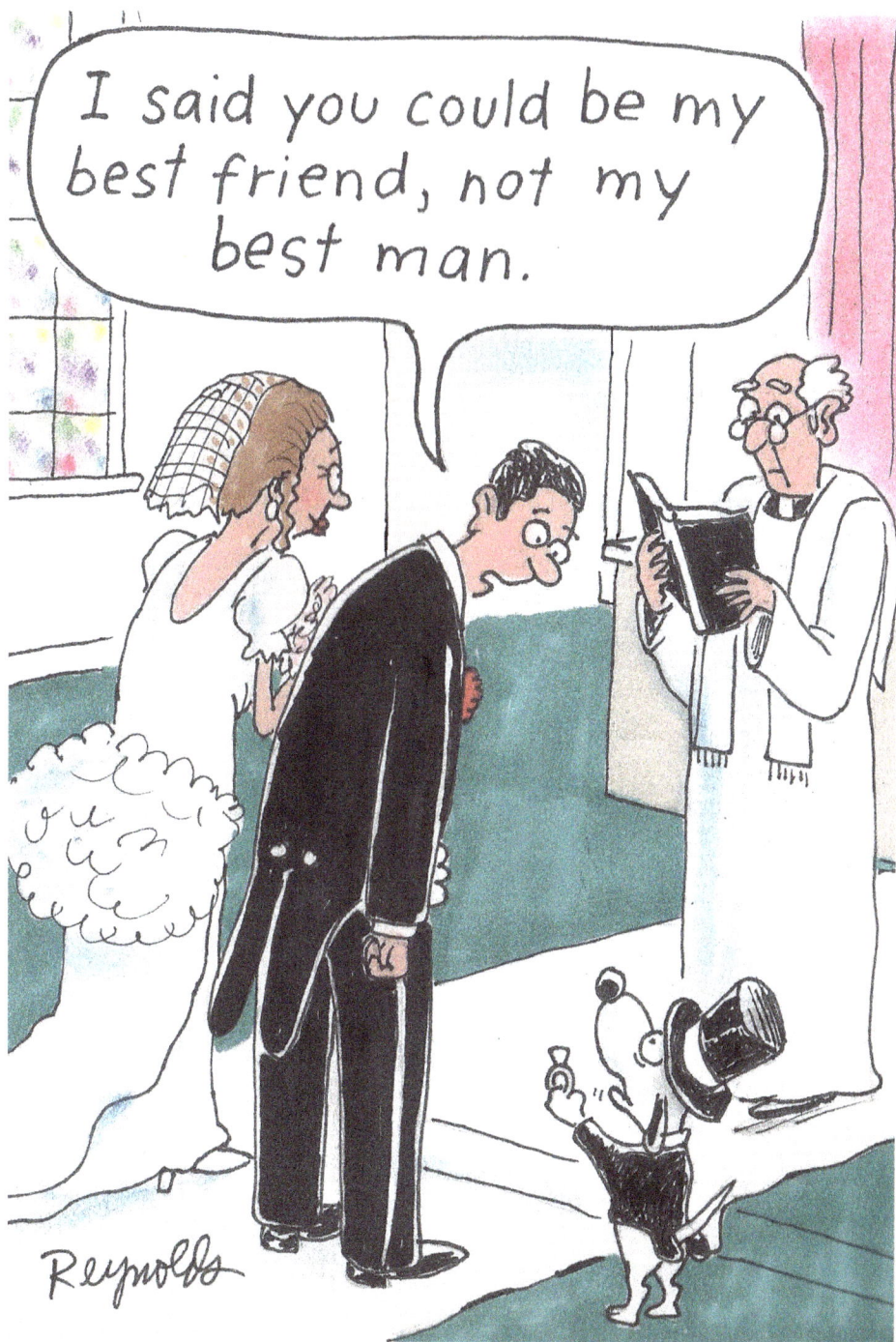

When dogs kick backward after they go to the bathroom it's not to cover it up, but to mark their territory, using the scent glands in their feet.

A recent study shows that dogs are among a small group of animals who show voluntary unselfish kindness towards others without any reward. This is one fact dog lovers have known all along.

The amount of money spent on dog food is 4 times as much as what is spent on baby food, 1.8 billion dollars.

The most common name for a dog is Max and while many people believe dogs sweat by panting this is not true—they sweat through the pads on their feet.

The Bible mentions dogs 14 times and the French Poodle did not originate in France.

The Bark Side: It's a Dog's Life!

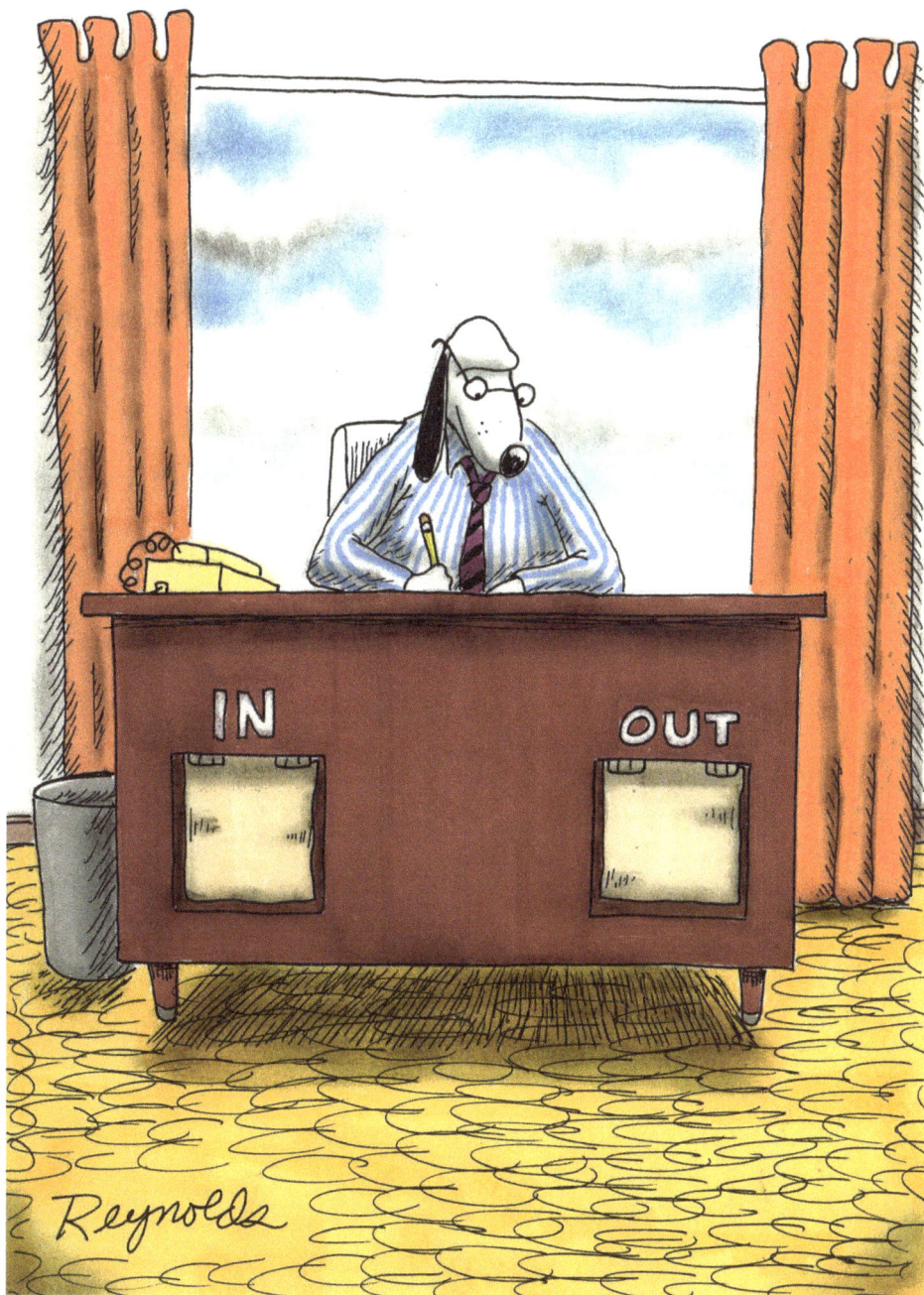

The Bark Side: It's a Dog's Life!

Dogs circle their bed several times before lying down. This goes back to when they were not yet domesticated. The dog would do this in the selected spot to check for snakes or other possible intruders. They also tend to lie with their nose to the wind as a precaution so their nose will pick up the scent of another animal or human moving towards them. They circle as a way to distribute their scent in the chosen spot and also a way to softens up the bedding spot.

Researchers have proven dogs can smell the presence of cancer in humans.

Research has shown people who own a dog live longer, have fewer hearts attacks, and have less daily stress.

Of all the breeds of dogs, only the Chow has a black tongue. All others are pink.

The Bark Side: It's a Dog's Life!

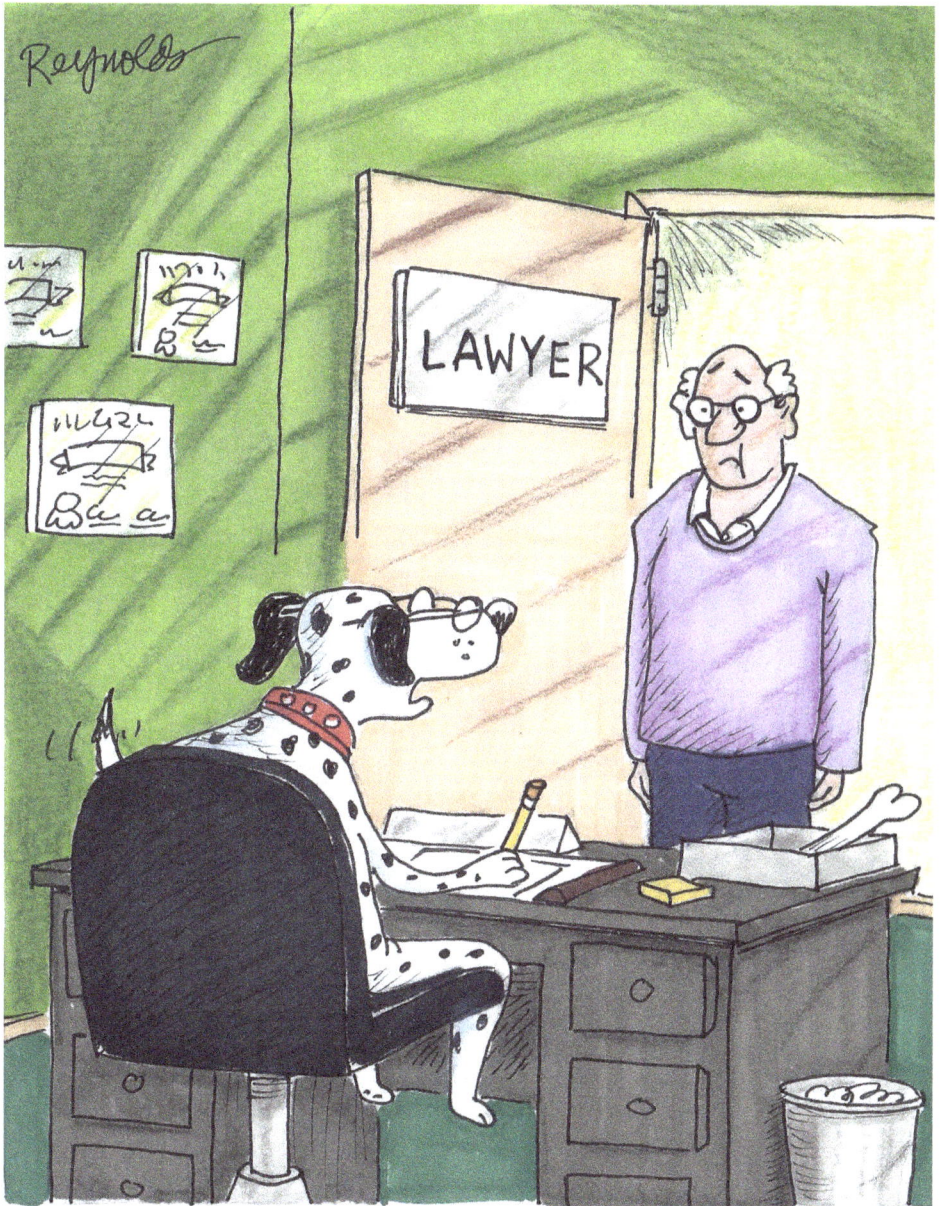

"Don't act so surprised. You're looking for an ambulance chaser, aren't you?"

The Bark Side: It's a Dog's Life!

96% of pet owners admit their dog brings a smile to their face at least once a day, while 33% talk to their dog on the phone as well as leaving messages on the answering machine for their dogs while they are away from home.

At least one million dog owners have made their dog the main beneficiary in their will.

The domestic dog (formally called *Canis lupus familiaris* or *Canis familiaris*) is a domesticated canid which performs many roles for people, such as hunting, herding, pulling loads, protection, assisting police and military, companionship and, more recently, aiding handicapped individuals. This influence on human society has given them the sobriquet, "man's best friend".

A male canine is referred to as a dog, while a female is called a bitch.

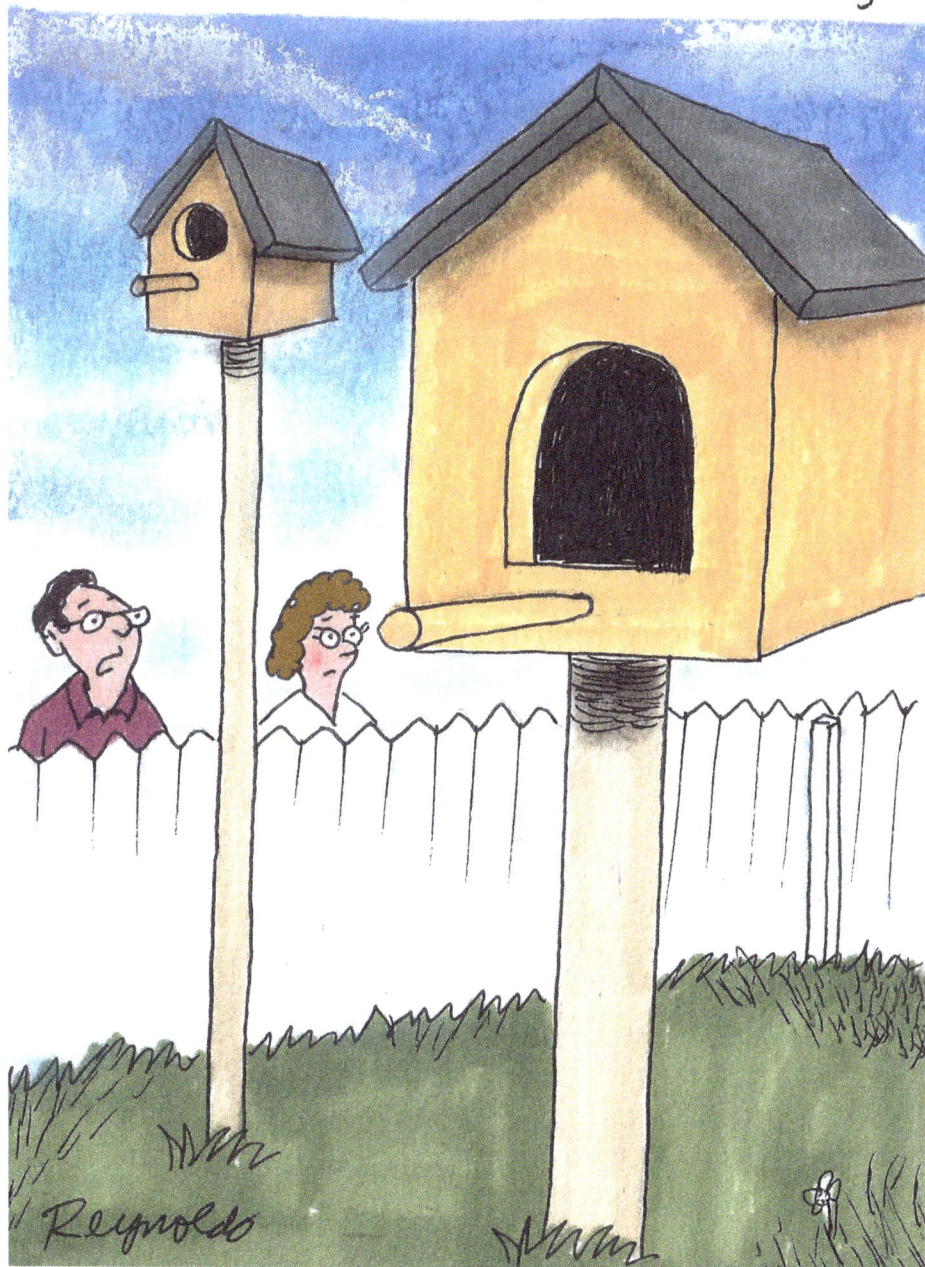

"The Capilli's just got a bird dog."

The Bark Side: It's a Dog's Life!

Extensive genetic studies undertaken during the 2010s indicate that dogs diverged from an extinct wolf-like canid in Eurasia 40,000 years ago

Their long association with humans has led to dogs being uniquely attuned to human behavior and are able to thrive on a starch-rich diet which would be inadequate for other canid species.

Dogs are also the oldest domesticated animal.

They vary widely in shape, size and colors.

In 14th-century England, hound was the general word for all domestic canines, and dog referred to a subtype of hound, a group including the mastiff. It is believed this "dog" type was so common, it eventually became the prototype of the category "hound".

The Bark Side: It's a Dog's Life!

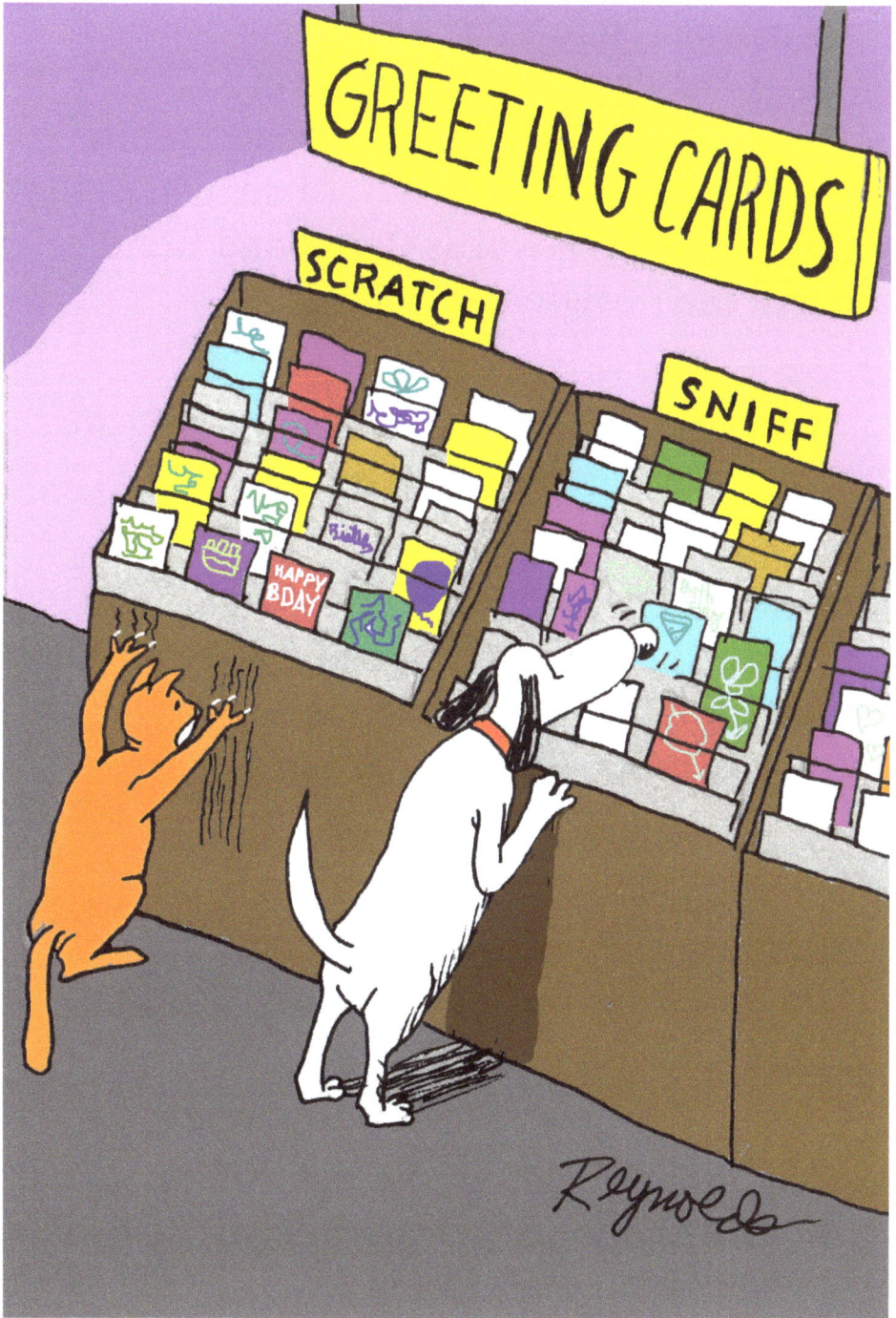

The Bark Side: It's a Dog's Life!

The word "hound" is ultimately derived from the Proto-Indo-European word *kwon-*, "dog". This semantic shift may be compared to in German, where the corresponding words Dogge and Hund kept their original meanings.

The father of a litter is called the sire, and the mother is called the dam.

A litter refers to the multiple offspring at one birth which are called puppies or pups from the French poupée, "doll", which has mostly replaced the older term "whelp".

Your dog is as smart as a 2-year-old toddler. They likely understand roughly the same number of words and gestures — 250!

Dogs do have better low-light vision than humans because of a special light-reflecting layer behind their retinas.

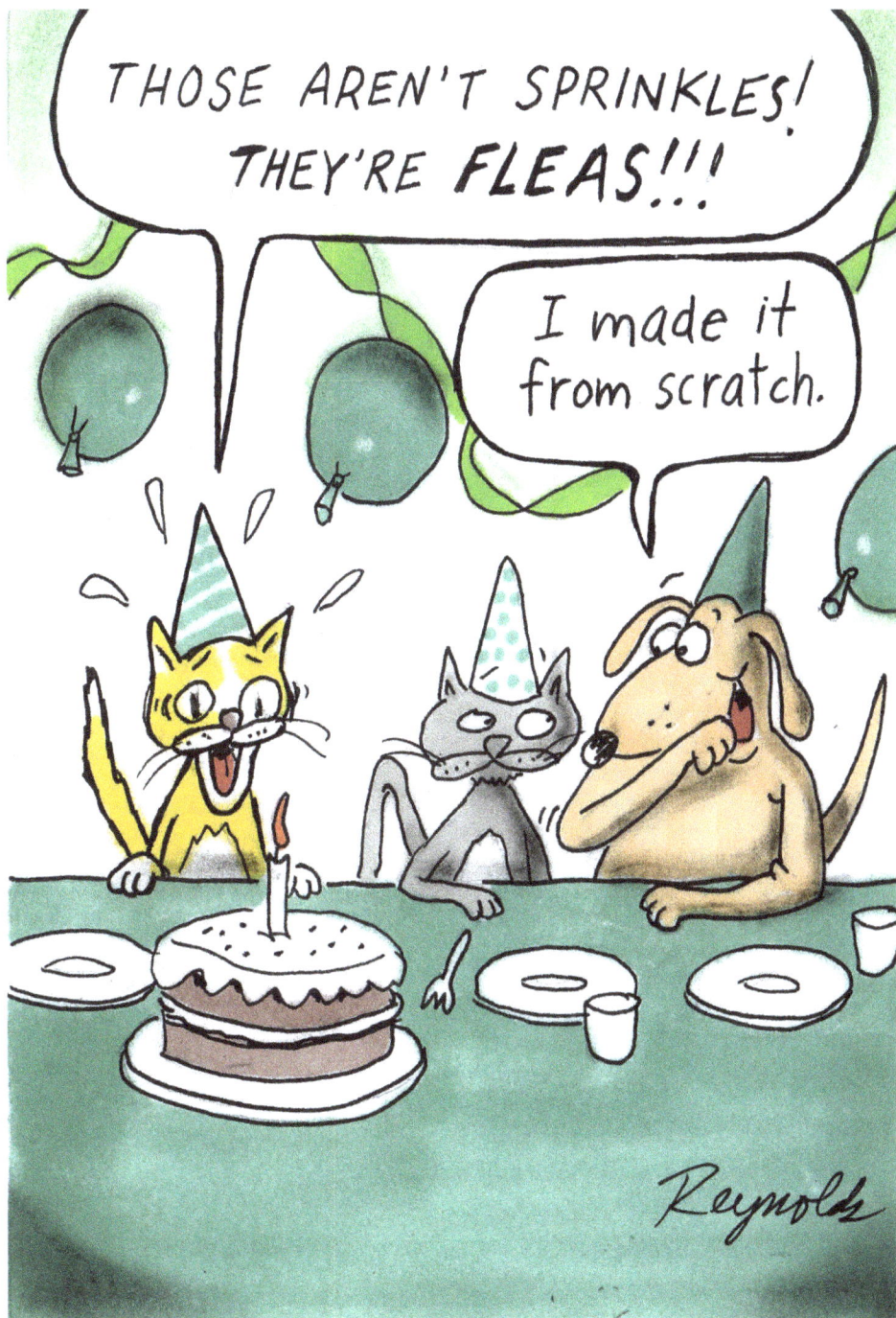

The Bark Side: It's a Dog's Life!

Dogs and cats both slurp water the same way. This may be hard to believe since dogs are such messy drinkers, but just like cats, our canine friends bend the tip of their tongue and raise liquid in a column up to their mouths.

When dogs kick after going to the bathroom, they are using the scent glands on their paws to further mark their territory.

Dogs can be trained to detect changes in the human body — there are even seizure alert dogs that assist patients during the onset of a seizure.

Labradors are the most popular breed in the United States.

It's a myth that dogs only see in black and white. In fact, it's believed that dogs see primarily in blue, greenish-yellow, yellow and various shades of gray.

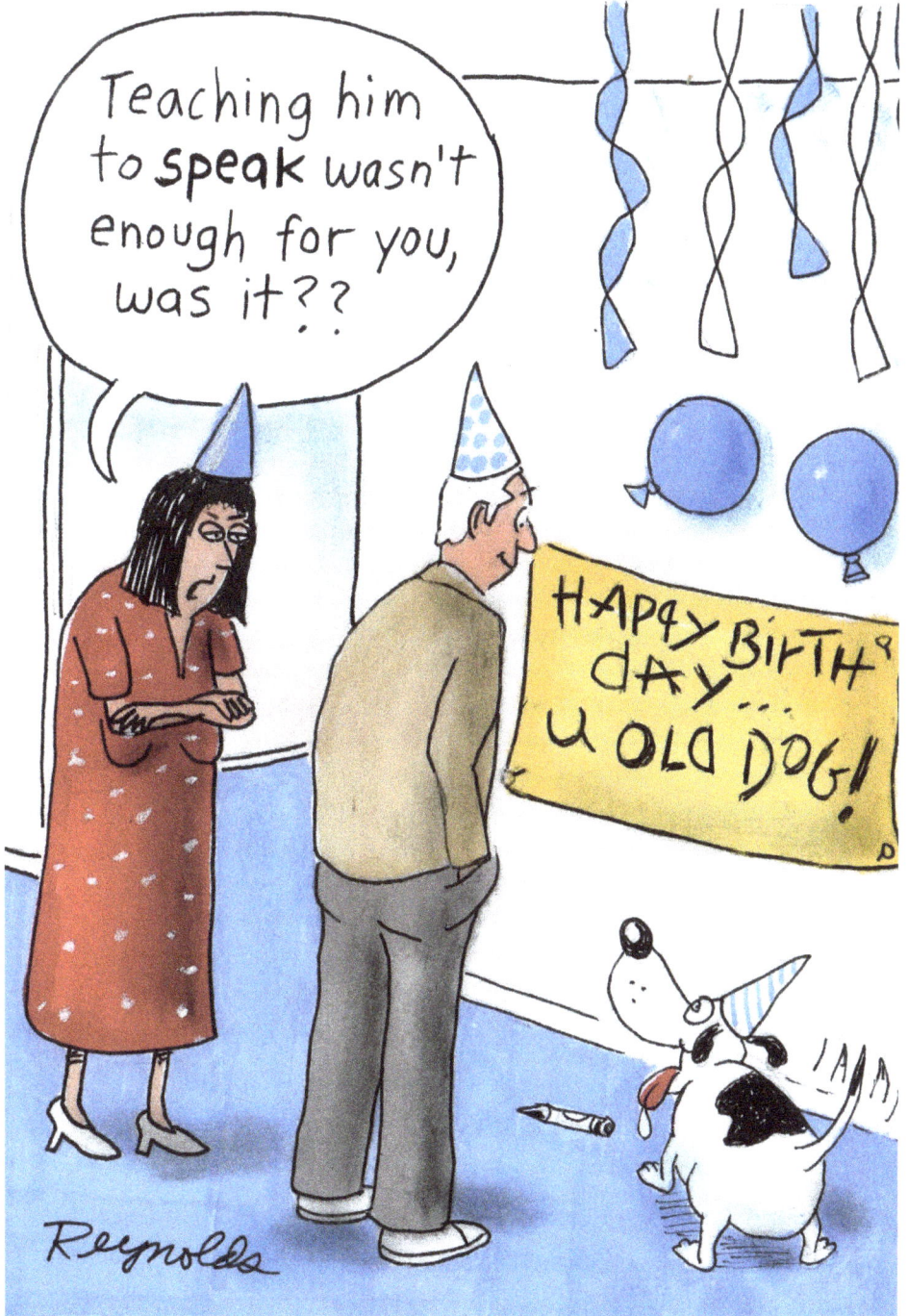

The Bark Side: It's a Dog's Life!

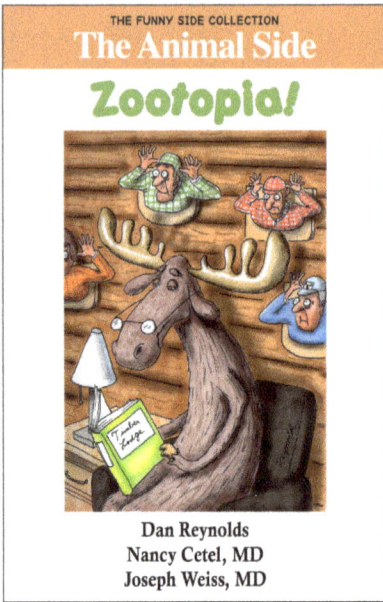

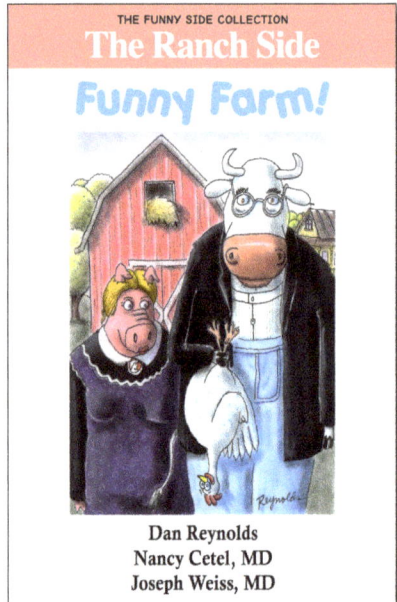

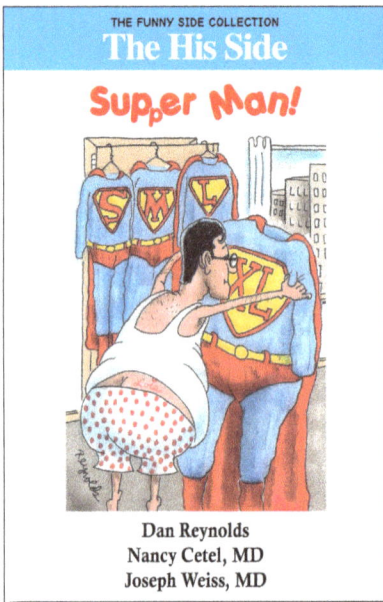

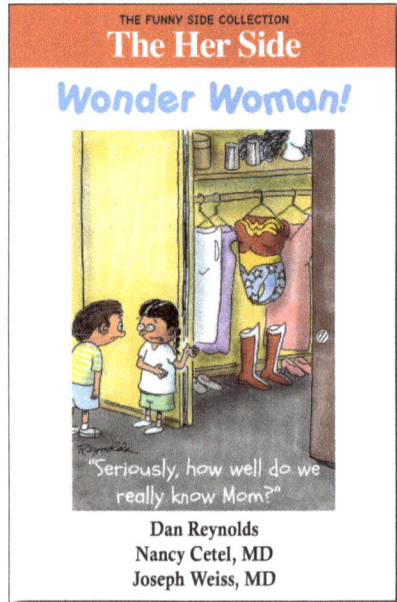

THE FUNNY SIDE COLLECTION
The Animal Side
Zootopia!

Dan Reynolds
Nancy Cetel, MD
Joseph Weiss, MD

THE FUNNY SIDE COLLECTION
The Ranch Side
Funny Farm!

Dan Reynolds
Nancy Cetel, MD
Joseph Weiss, MD

THE FUNNY SIDE COLLECTION
The His Side
Supper Man!

Dan Reynolds
Nancy Cetel, MD
Joseph Weiss, MD

THE FUNNY SIDE COLLECTION
The Her Side
Wonder Woman!

"Seriously, how well do we really know Mom?"

Dan Reynolds
Nancy Cetel, MD
Joseph Weiss, MD

www.thefunnysidecollection.com

The Bark Side: It's a Dog's Life!

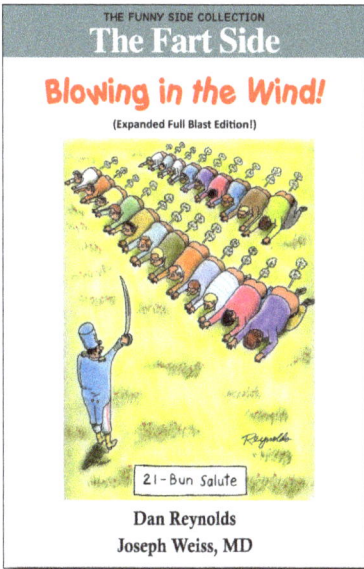

THE FUNNY SIDE COLLECTION
The Fart Side
Blowing in the Wind!
(Expanded Full Blast Edition!)
21-Bun Salute
Dan Reynolds
Joseph Weiss, MD

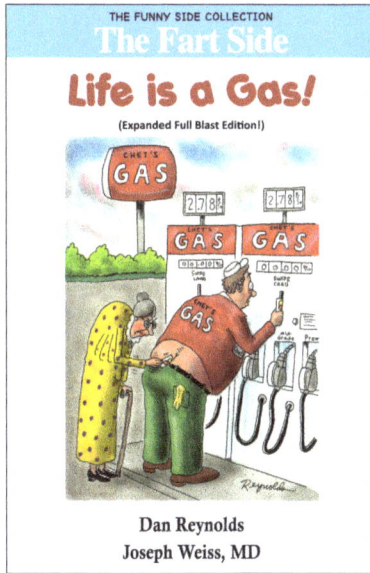

THE FUNNY SIDE COLLECTION
The Fart Side
Life is a Gas!
(Expanded Full Blast Edition!)
Dan Reynolds
Joseph Weiss, MD

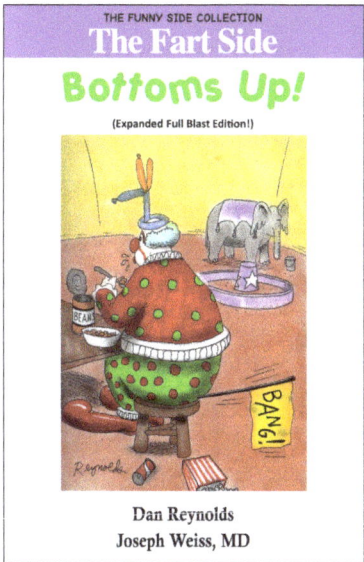

THE FUNNY SIDE COLLECTION
The Fart Side
Bottoms Up!
(Expanded Full Blast Edition!)
Dan Reynolds
Joseph Weiss, MD

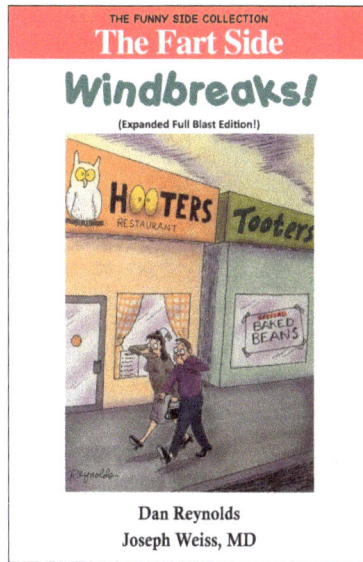

THE FUNNY SIDE COLLECTION
The Fart Side
Windbreaks!
(Expanded Full Blast Edition!)
Dan Reynolds
Joseph Weiss, MD

Available in 5"x7" (96 pages) Pocket Rocket! & 6"x9" (122 pages) Expanded Full Blast! print/e-book edition

www.thefunnysidecollection.com

The Bark Side: It's a Dog's Life!

Dan Reynolds

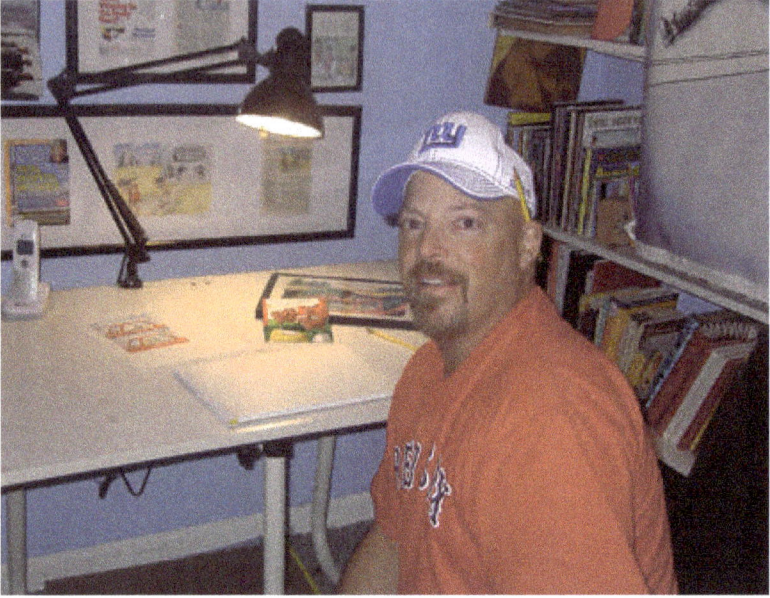

Dan Reynolds began drawing cartoons in December of 1989. He draws and eats left-handed. He plays ping pong and pool left-handed. He throws, kicks and bats right-handed. Like a box of chocolates, you never know what you're going to get, but you will like most of them and they'll keep you coming back. Unlike chocolates, REYNOLDS UNWRAPPED cartoons are not fattening.

Dan's cartoons are seen by millions of readers across the US, Canada and points beyond all the way down under in Australia. His work is seen in every issue of Reader's Digest (where he is known for his cow, pig and chicken cartoons), on greetings cards everywhere. His cartoons have appeared on HBO's, The Sopranos, the cover of a National Lampoon cartoon book collection

The Bark Side: It's a Dog's Life!

and on greeting cards all throughout the United States. His work also appears in many other places as well.

Sign-up for Dan's daily REYNOLDS UNWRAPPED e-mail cartoon for only $12 for a whole year. E-mail Dan at reynoldsunwrapped@gmail.com for details. Dan's website is:

www.reynoldsunwrapped.weebly.com

The Funny Side Collection, The Fart Side series, and other items are available at:

www.smartaskbooks.com
www.thefunnysidecollection.com

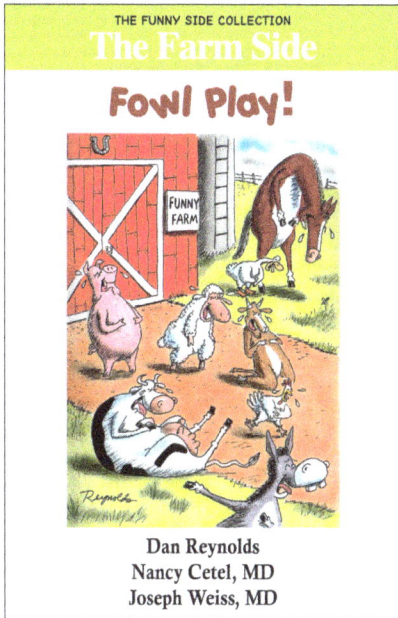

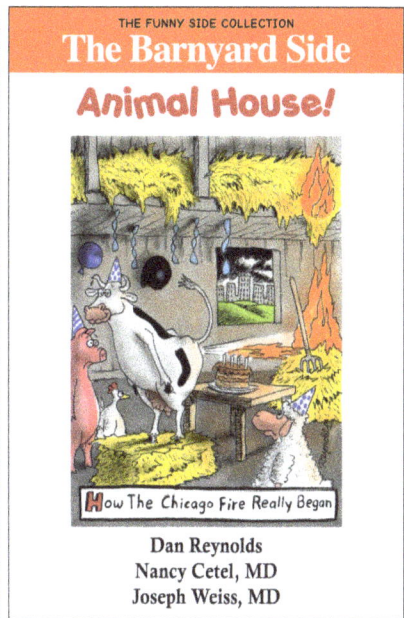

www.thefunnysidecollection.com

The Bark Side: It's a Dog's Life!

Nancy Cetel, M.D.

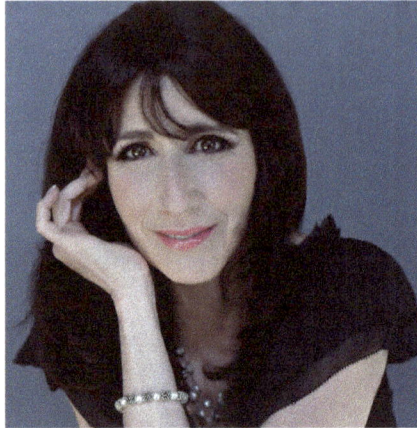

Nancy Cetel, MD is an engaging and passionate physician, educator, author, professional speaker, and humorist. She has given hundreds of presentations, with the audiences ranging from medical professors and professionals to sophisticated lay audiences. Live appearances and interviews before local, regional, national and International television and radio audiences have brought her acclaim as an accomplished communicator and advocate for an informed public.

As a Future Farmer of America (FFA) her career path was leading to veterinary medicine, but human medicine intervened. Following her graduation from the New York University School of Medicine, she traveled to the West Coast where she obtained her postgraduate training in Obstetrics and Gynecology at The University of California, and University of Southern California. She also served on the faculty of the University of California where she completed an additional three years of postgraduate training in Reproductive Endocrinology.

Her pioneering research led to numerous publications and awards including the lead article in the prestigious New England Journal of Medicine. Dr. Cetel has been in medical practice in California for over twenty-five years, and maintains a keen interest in preventive health care, hormonal balance, and age management medicine. She has had numerous publications in prestigious medical and lay journals and magazines.

As a distinguished former academic researcher and clinician, she undertook the writing of the groundbreaking book, Double Menopause: What to do When You and Your Mate go Through Hormonal Changes Together, dealing with midlife hormonal issues for men and women. Dr. Cetel is often referenced in books and journals, and is a frequently invited lecturer nationally and internationally. Her passions include her family, vegetarian cooking, tap dancing, and the joys of being a grandparent.

Dr. Cetel is a frequently invited professional speaker and humorist, at universities, international conventions, conferences, corporations, resorts, and special events with programs that exemplify edutainment. She is the author of several dozen books and articles on health available at:

www.smartaskbooks.com and
www.doublemenopause.com

The Bark Side: It's a Dog's Life!

The Funny Side Collection, The Fart Side series, and other items are available at:

www.thefunnysidecollection.com

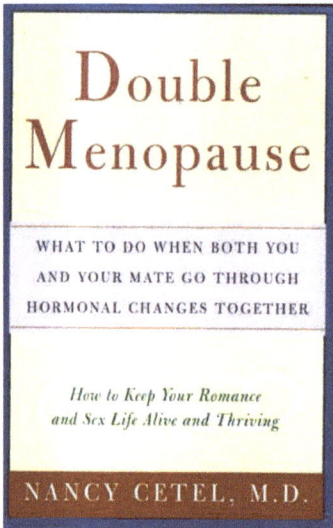

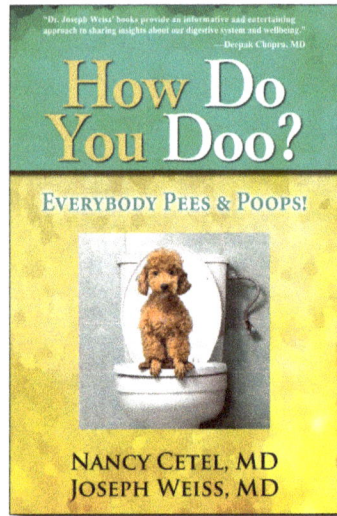

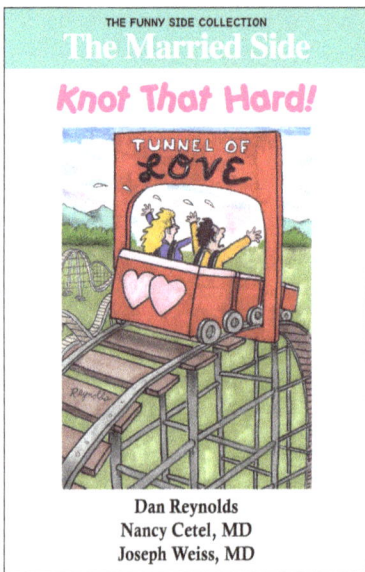

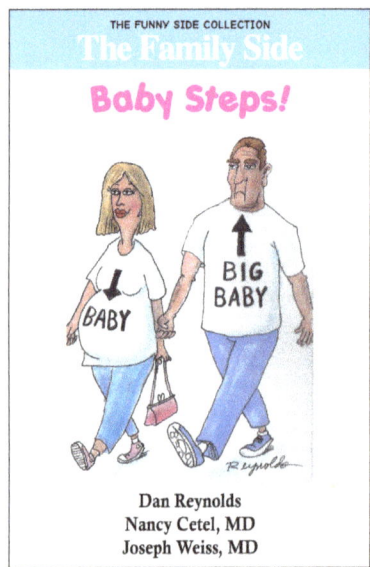

www.doublemenopause.com
www.smartaskbooks.com

The Bark Side: It's a Dog's Life!

Joseph Weiss, M.D.

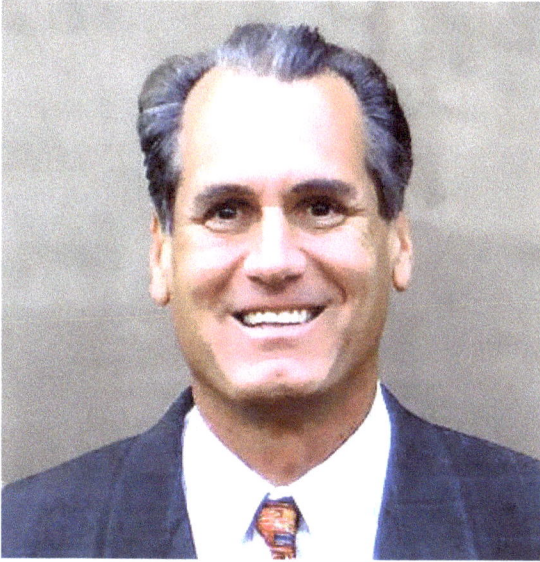

GI Joe is Clinical Professor of Medicine in the Division of Gastroenterology at the University of California, San Diego. He is a Fellow of the American College of Physicians, American Gastroenterological Association, and American College of Gastroenterology.

He is an accomplished professional speaker and humorist, having given over three thousand invited presentations internationally at universities, international conventions, conferences, corporations, resorts, and special events. Dr. Weiss is the author of several dozen books on health available at:

www.smartaskbooks.com

The Funny Side Collection, The Fart Side series, and other items are available at:

www.thefunnysidecollection.com

The Bark Side: It's a Dog's Life!

"Dr. Joseph Weiss' books provide an informative and entertaining approach to sharing insights about our digestive system and wellbeing." **Deepak Chopra, MD**

"Joseph Weiss, M.D. has a gift for books that are uniquely informative and entertaining." **Jack Canfield** Coauthor of the *Chicken Soup for the Soul®* series

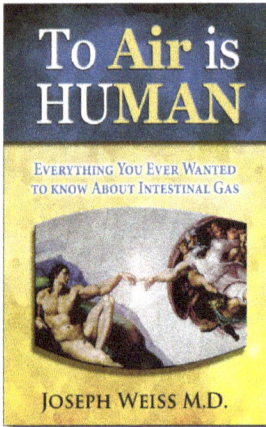

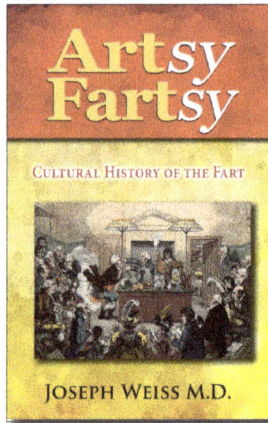

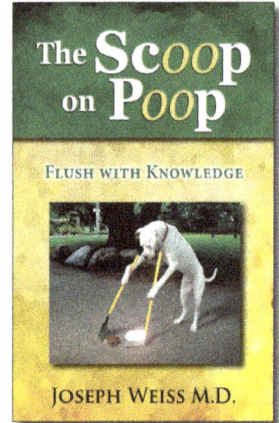

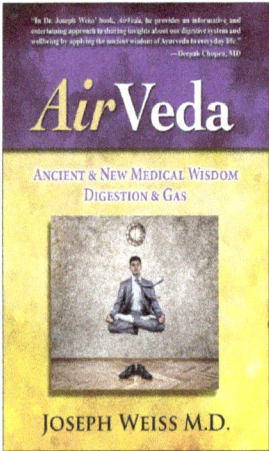

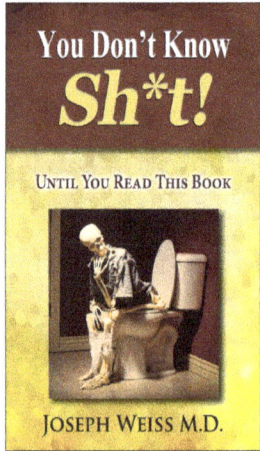

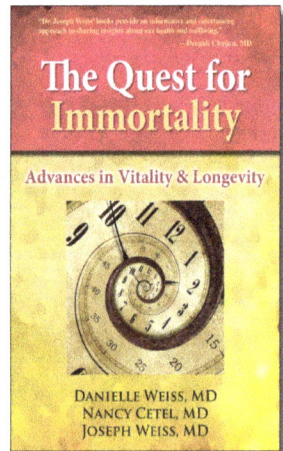

www.smartaskbooks.com
www.thefunnysidecollection.com

www.ingramcontent.com/pod-product-compliance
Lightning Source LLC
Chambersburg PA
CBHW051247020426

42333CB00025B/3091